FAT FREE
FOREVER

BOBBY RAY

FAT FREE FOREVER

Copyright © 2008 by Bobby Ray
ISBN 978-1-59712-312-9

Acknowledgments

I want to give special thanks to the following people without whom the publication of this book would not have been possible:

Mary C. Ray
Members of Assembly Faith Church and Ministry Partners
Pastor Dean Melton of Freedom Christian Center
Andrew Wommack
My daughter Melissa Elders
Roberta Dawson

To Cathy Ray, my wife of thirty-two years, whom I love and cherish very deeply. Your encouragement and help made this book possible. Thank you for loving me and standing by me through "thick and thin."

Contents

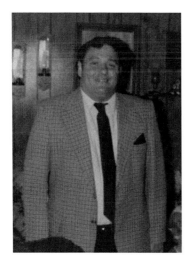
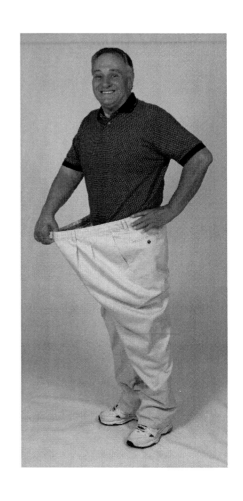
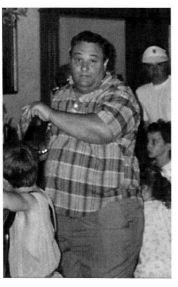
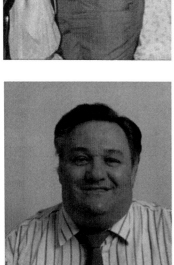
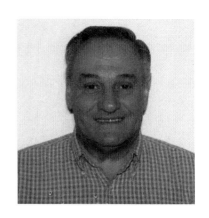

My Story

Overeating was always a problem for me. My problem began when I was very young. I did not start being excessively overweight until I was about twelve years old. But even before age twelve, I remember overeating being a part of my life. Friday was grocery day at our house and it was like a celebration to me. I would eat five banana sandwiches, cookies, and drink three glasses of milk. I ate so much, not because we didn't have enough to eat at our house, but because I remember something inside saying to me, "You better eat some more." These thoughts gave me reasons to overeat, believing that I would somehow miss out on the foods I liked. I remember when my mom would bake a cake and I would eat two large pieces of cake and then sneak back into the kitchen when no one was looking and get two more.

Throughout my whole life I made wrong choices, eating different types of foods. I played a lot of sports: baseball, football, and basketball. Although I stayed very active through high school I remember that I didn't lose weight during football practices, because I still over ate as much as possible. Even when I was full, I would convince myself to eat more. I got to the point of being a sugar addict, eating sweets all the time. Thoughts of food and sweets were constantly on my mind.

When I got drafted into the U.S. Army at age eighteen, I was thirty-five pounds overweight. I went through basic training and two years of service but still gained twenty pounds. Twenty pounds may not seem like a lot to you; but it is, especially when you add the thirty-five pounds I had already gained. I remember going to a naval base for three days. They told us, "Eat all you want, but do not waste." So on the first day for breakfast, I ate six eggs, four biscuits, four boxes of sweet cereal, milk, coffee, and dessert. I didn't eat all of this because I was hungry or because I wanted all of it. I ate it because it was available. As you can see, I definitely had a major problem with overeating.

I came out of the army 55 pounds overweight. Shortly after I was released from the service there was a six-year period in my life when I was not overweight, and this was due to sickness. Because of the medications I was taking, I lost my appetite. My weight dropped down to 145 pounds. After I got well from the sickness, the battle in my mind continued. I gained back my weight and much more, tipping the scale at 300 pounds! At the time, my parents owned a restaurant and I worked there. I was faced with temptation constantly. I felt compelled to eat. So instead of being tormented, I gave in over and over again. I went with the flow: eat, eat, eat.

After being healed, I gained over 155 pounds. We would go to a fish camp and I would eat more than three times what the average person would, getting reorders of french fries, hushpuppies and even eating other people's food. I remember our family and friends going to McDonald's. I would eat my food and my family's, and wish they would offer me more. I would go pick up food to take home and eat some off of each plate, and I still ate the biggest order. I weighed 300 pounds and saw no end in sight. I ate six sweets a day: ice cream, cake, cookies and sodas.

But then I found the truth and lost 110 pounds. I went from a size 50 pant to a size 34. I went from a 3X shirt to a normal large or medium. So it really is an honor and privilege to be sharing these truths concerning weight reduction with you.

Anyone can do what I did and lose that much weight. You can do it if you follow the simple instructions and truths of this book.

Not only did I get rid of 110 pounds but I've kept it off. Look at my picture below and see how far I've come from the way I was before. Wrong eating will never be a problem for me again! I have the key to victory. I can go to any restaurant with my family now and still do not eat the wrong things. It does not bother me. I am free! Absolutely free! Totally unrestrained, and I have absolutely no pressure, none whatsoever.

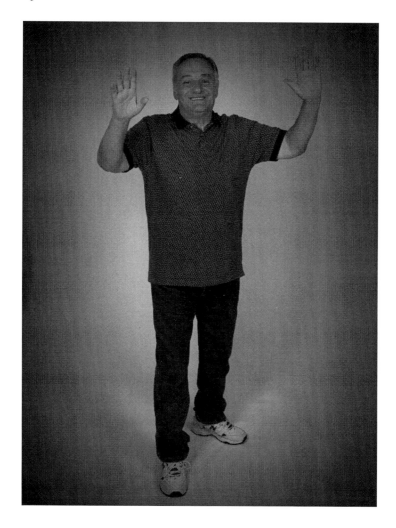

Definitions of Words

I want to give you definitions of different words I will use throughout the book. If you understand the definitions of these words, they will bring more light and you will have more understanding concerning the way things work.

Word

What does it mean when you hear "word?" What is it all about? Simply put, a word is a seed and you must always know it is a seed. Anywhere a seed is planted in good ground it always brings forth a good harvest. You don't ever have to make a seed reproduce; all you have to do is plant it in the ground. In fact, seeds have been known to spring forth from between cracks in concrete, and also in rocks. A seed is very powerful.

Seeds can be planted in two ways: through hearing and through speaking. Both ways are interrelated in that they are always present with each other. If someone is speaking, someone is also hearing, and vice-versa. The way you plant seeds is by speaking them out of your mouth. Once you speak a word out of your mouth, a seed is planted. Understand that.

Seeds Have an Image

So with that in mind also understand that every seed has an image or blueprint of itself on the inside of it. A small orange seed has the blueprint of orange tree on the inside of it. However, the image is so tiny that if you would cut that seed open you could not see that orange tree. This image or blueprint can also be called DNA. When creating the world, God said, *Let the earth bring forth grass, the herb yielding seed, and the fruit tree yielding fruit after his kind, whose seed is in itself, upon the earth: and it was so. And the earth brought forth grass, and herb yielding seed after his kind, and the tree yielding fruit, whose seed was in itself, after his kind: and God saw that it was good.* [Genesis 1:11-12]

Every seed has an image of itself on the inside of it and it grows or reproduces the image that's on the inside of the seed. It does it automatically. You don't have to make it do it, it will automatically do it. All you have to do is to plant the seed and take care of the seed that is planted, and it will bring forth a crop. It is impossible for a seed to not bring forth a crop if you plant it and take care of it.

So with that in mind, every word is filled with the stuff (or elements) of the meaning of that word. For example, water has the elements hydrogen and oxygen. Salt has sodium and chlorine. Each word is filled with elements that are words as well. Every word is filled or has an image of the elements of the meaning of that word. It's important that you know this.

Something Spoken

Another simple meaning of the word "word" or "words" is something said or spoken. When you are speaking words you are computing and calculating the results of what is going to happen. *God said, Let there be light: and there was light.* [Genesis 1:3] Therefore, God spoke for a purpose of accomplishing something.

Calculation of Results

Word also refers to computing or calculation of results. A result is computed according to the amount of seeds that were sown. For instance, if you planted one row of corn, then you can only reap a harvest of one row of corn. If you sowed fifty acres of corn, then you have the potential to reap fifty acres of corn because that is what you sowed. That seed will automatically compute the results. You don't have to make the results happen.

I want to remind you that all you have to do is sow the word or the words and it will automatically compute the results for you according to the meaning of that word. I think that is very good, and God said this process was good (Genesis 1:12).

Let's say that I planted words, and based on this principle, they will automatically bring results. Therefore, when you continue to tell yourself that you do not like certain kinds of foods like granulated sugar, and foods like that are not good for you, those words will automatically go to your soul (mind, will and emotions) and they will compute to your taste buds and after a period of time they will tell you that you do not like sugar anymore. Using the power of words as seeds, you don't have to make yourself quit eating sugar. If you continue speaking words to that effect, it won't be long until you will not even want it. It's much easier to quit something that you don't like or don't want anymore than it is to try and quit something that you still want or crave.

Communication

Another part or element of the word "words" is communication. That's what words do, they communicate. We can understand very easily that words communicate because if I want to talk to you or communicate something to you I use words in a conversation, and I get my point across to you. Is that right? You also use words to communicate to yourself. Words that you speak also communicate to you. So you can take words that are spoken and since communication is an element of "words" therefore you can communicate to yourself what you want.

You Are What You Say

You are the sum total of the words you have heard and spoken. Barring the fact that there might be something wrong in your body that could cause it, the reason you are overweight today is because you have told yourself that you like certain kinds of foods that you should not be eating and therefore you continue to eat them.

It is easy to get rid of excess weight when you no longer like the foods that are bad for you. It is not hard. It is the act of transmitting. When you're speaking words you're transmitting things—information, sending signals. You're sending messages. I want you to get a hold of this. When you're speaking words you are transmitting information, sending signals and messages to your mind, will and emotions. So if you send the right signals, and transmit the right things to your mind, will and emotions, then it will cause you to think differently and you know that the way we think is the way we will live.

Intent or Purpose

Another element of the word "word" is intent. Intent causes you to have a fixed result. It will affect the mind and the attention span, and it will strongly resolve situations in your life. It will affect the purpose of one's mental attitude. In other words, you don't have to make words affect the purpose of your mental attitude. They will automatically affect the purpose of your mental attitude. Intent includes purpose and will cause you to have determination to reach your goal of getting rid of excess weight off your body.

You have to understand that you don't have to make words work for you; all you have to do is plant them and continue to water them by repeating them and they will automatically work for you. The purpose or intent of what you are speaking is already programmed into the word to achieve the expected results. Words will relate the information to your mind, will and emotions and they will begin to change your mind. You will begin to wash your mind with the water of those words, and you will actually begin to brainwash or re-wash your mind with right thinking. That's exactly what will happen. It's not bad to brainwash yourself as long as if it's good clean water (words). Wash your thinking with the good, healthy, and beneficial words of God.

Power

Another element of a word is "power." God's word tells us in Proverbs 18:21 that there is power in words. *Death and life are in the power of the tongue: and they that love it shall eat the fruit thereof.*

There is inherent power in words; and there is already power inside of those words to accomplish what those words are about or what those words mean. The word power refers to ability. So we understand here that because there is power in words, we are able to accomplish whatever we speak. As a matter of fact, the second meaning of the word power is to accomplish. The meaning of the word "power" is the ability to produce or to do. It is the ability to carry it out. Now understand again that power is on the inside of words and this is the meaning of the word "power".

When the angel Gabriel told Mary, *For with God nothing shall be impossible* [Luke 1:37] he was actually saying, "No word of God is without power, strength, or ability of fulfillment."

Power means specified ability according to what words you are using. It means great ability to do it. Can you see from these meanings that you do not have to struggle over excess weight on your body or anything else that's a hindrance to you? You do not have to struggle for the rest of your life getting rid of five, ten, or twenty pounds and then gain it back. Can you see that by proper speaking of words and the power that's in those words, that it will automatically cause you to be free?

I'm going to tell you once again that I got rid of over 100

pounds by this method. I did not take pills. I did not mix up a powder. I did not come up with some kind of gimmick. I didn't come up with a certain kind of formula. I didn't have to have an operation. I didn't have to have my stomach stapled, or something tied to keep me feeling full and curb my desire to eat. I didn't do any of that. I didn't have to eat twelve grapefruits a day. Or the one where you eat bananas all day one day, and eat oranges the next, and apples the next day. There's nothing wrong with eating those foods. I'm just talking about the methods people use to lose weight. But did you ever notice that the majority of people who lose weight always gain it back? After losing it, they seem to always find it. So this book is not about losing weight; it's about getting rid of excess weight off of you body forever. That's the key; it's forever.

Specified Ability

Part of the meaning of the word "power" is a specified ability. It is great ability to do, to carry it out, to accomplish, and to complete it. It means to be strong. It means to have vigor. It means to have force. It means to have strength. It means to have the ability to sway yourself, to control yourself and to influence yourself.

In the beginning, these words and the power in these words will begin to sway you. They will begin to influence you, and they will change your mind. They'll change your mind and give you the power; and later you will use this same power to influence others.

Authority

Another meaning of the word "power" is authority. One reason why most people fail when they go on a certain kind of a diet, and they give up on it is because of authority. You haven't been able to get rid of excess weight off your body in the past because you have not taken authority over your issue of getting rid of excess weight.

Inherent Ability

Another meaning of the word "power" is inherent ability. It is the admitted right to rule and govern your own life. When you have power, you have inherent ability, the admitted right to rule and govern your own life. Having power means that you have the ability to restrain and curb yourself.

Another meaning of the word "power" is the ability, force and freedom. Isn't freedom a powerful word? Freedom is miracle working power.

Life

The next word I want to give you the meaning of is life. Life refers to living, being; alive, afresh, anew; living the right kind of life. Life is not being tormented by excess weight on your body and thinking you can't get rid of it, but knowing now that you can and you will get rid of it. Words have power that produce life. Death and life are in the power of words.

Mouth

The next word I want to give you the meaning of is the word "mouth." Mouth is a powerful word and if you look it up in the Greek it means a gash in the face, an opening in the earth. But on the spiritual side it means the front edge as of a weapon. Now you can take the front edge of a weapon and you can destroy your enemy, which is excess weight, and eating wrong foods. You can destroy your enemy with it or you can take that weapon and you can harm yourself. Anyone knows that if someone attacks you, you can use a knife or gun to defend yourself. But on the other hand, if you use that knife or gun improperly, you could hurt or kill your own self. Do you see what I'm saying?

What I'm telling you is to take proper words and speak them over yourself; talk to yourself about them, and use your mouth, the front edge of that weapon, to destroy your enemy—excess weight.

How many of you know that when something is destroyed it dies? It has to leave. It can't hang around any longer. Is that your goal? Is your objective that your excess weight will leave forever?

Tongue

Now I want to move to the meaning of the word "tongue". Tongue is a powerful word. In the natural it means a source of lapping. The tongue is a source of lapping like a dog or a person got down and just lapped water with it. But let me tell you what it means in the spirit. The meaning of the word tongue in the spiritual realm is wedge. What do you do with a wedge? You take a wedge and you drive it into something to separate those things. A wedge is used to remove one side from the other side. So when you use your tongue by speaking proper words, you drive a wedge in between you and wrong eating habits, which brought wrong results of excess weight on your body.

Now let me stress something to you here. Wishing excess weight would leave your body won't make it leave. I know because I wished it to leave my body for years and years. Crying over it will not make it leave your body, I know because I've cried over it. Hoping alone will not make it leave your body. You have to do something about it. And the way that I'm telling you to do something about it, is to get the job done. Make the excess weight leave by doing it the right and proper way, not through a gimmick and not even being tormented over it.

The word "free" means to be totally unrestrained. It means when you're totally free, you're free to walk away from it, to not look back and not be tormented by it at all. That's what I call being free from excess weight. That is what I call being free from wrong eating habits. That's what I call being free. In other words, you're totally unrestrained. Those wrong foods do not bother you anymore. You walk away from them and they are no longer a part of your life and you're not even tempted by them anymore.

Think

Now I want to talk to you about the word "think". I want to give you a couple of quick definitions of the word think. The word "think" means to think. How do you like that? That was a great revelation, wasn't it? It also means to ponder. In other words, it means to study it through, to meditate on it. If you're going to think something through or think it out, you're going to spend a little time with it. The word "think" and the word "thought" are two different words. They do join each other at one point down the road, but they do not mean the same exact thing. A thought can be just a fleeting thought that passes through your mind. If you do not give considerable thinking, pondering and meditating on that thought, then you have not moved into the realm of thinking about it. Do you understand what I'm saying? It takes some time. You've got to ponder it to think about it. You've got to meditate on it a while to think about it.

Now let me tell you the spiritual meaning of the word "think". It means to open. Every single thing that you think, ponder, and meditate on, you open yourself to. So when you speak the proper words, telling yourself that you do not like the taste of granulated sugar anymore, and you do like the taste of other things that are good for you, you take a minute to think, and it opens you up to these things. As the old saying goes, use your head for something else other than a hat rack. Think, ponder, and meditate. And when you open yourself to right and proper thoughts, you will have what you say.

Soul

The next word I want to go over with you is the word "soul". The soul consists of the mind, the will, and the emotions. Every person is a three-dimensional being: You are a spirit; you possess a soul, which is your mind, will, and emotions; and you live in a physical body, which includes the five senses that dominate your physical life. Every word you hear or speak is a seed. And every one of these seeds and all that they contain are planted in your soul. They are planted and they affect your mind. They affect the way you begin to think. They affect the way you begin to talk after a period of time. They affect your mind and your will.

When your will begins to be affected, then you begin to will or desire to do these things. Once you will to do the right thing, it becomes much easier. Once you persuade your will to get in line with what you desire in your heart, then you begin to affect the emotional realm. When you begin to affect the emotional realm, you will cause motion. That is what will finally drive you to get rid of that excess weight and live a healthier lifestyle. Because we all know, that when we get rid of excess weight from our bodies, we become healthier. Getting rid of excess weight forever causes us to live a longer life than we would have lived otherwise.

Images
The next word that I want to talk to you about is "images." You create images or pictures on the inside of your mind. Once you build the picture or the image of seeing yourself eating proper foods and not eating improper foods, then it becomes very easy to carry it out. I want to make this as simple as possible. If you begin to train your mind, will, and emotions before you get started on the new way of eating and the proper diet plan, and you prepare yourself for it, then it makes it much easier and not difficult at all to take care of.

chapter
1
What is a Diet?

Most people when they hear the word "diet" they automatically think, "Oh no, diet? I'm not going on another diet. I'll have to quit eating this or I'll have to quit eating that or I'll have to start doing this or I'll have to start doing that."

But a diet simply means the plan that you use to live by each and every day. Let's look at the meaning of diet, and this will become real to you. You're going to find out that the word diet is really not a bad word. Neither is it really anything to be afraid of. A diet is something you experience every day in your life. You're on a diet right now, because one definition of diet is simply what a person eats and/or drinks regularly.

Webster's Dictionary has several definitions of the word "diet." Have you ever heard anyone argue with Webster's Dictionary? The first meaning of the word diet is "daily food allowance." All of us have a daily food allowance, don't we? Every one of us have a daily food allowance. The difference is what we choose to spend the daily allowance on.

The next meaning of diet is "way of life." All of us have a way of life. Another definition of diet is "what a person usually eats or drinks regularly." All of us eat and drink different things regularly. Webster's also refers to diet as, "what a person reads and listens to." I want you to see this so I'm going to repeat it: a diet is what a person reads and listens to.

The final definition of diet is one most people associate with the word: "a special or limited amount of food and drink chosen or prescribed to promote health, to gain weight, or the loss of weight; to eat or cause to eat special or limited foods for losing weight."

Did you notice that word special in there? When you follow a diet program properly you are now special. You'll begin to feel better about yourself; you'll see that you really are special. Something special is deep inside you and you didn't even know it. A diet is "to eat or cause to eat special or limited foods for losing weight." We are not deprived; we are special. Just because we are

Webster's also refers to diet as, "what a person reads and listens to."

changing some of the areas of our diet plan does not mean we are deprived at all. It means that we are now special, that we are able to choose our food and drink properly. That sounds good, doesn't it? It's not hard to choose. You have the right to choose. You don't have to be dictated by all of the foods that have controlled you thus far in your life. You no longer have to be controlled by them. You can control what you choose to eat to lose weight.

It's amazing how much Webster's Dictionary not only gives us the facts concerning the word diet but it brings truth into this area. Once you see the truth and wisdom of doing this my way, weight loss will be very easy for you. I want to break down the word diet so that you can totally understand it.

The dictionary says that a diet is a way of life. What's a "way of life?" The word "way" means "to go, means of travel, to go from one point to another, means of passing from one place to another, as a road, a highway or a street." Can you see the meaning of the word way? It is like a highway or a route you are choosing each and every day in your life to travel from one point to another point.

Therefore, a diet is a highway, a road or a path. A diet is a free area, an opening. This is what you will be creating, an opening where you can move freely without strain to your destination of weight reduction. Remember we are describing the word "diet."

We are talking about weight reduction and I'm going to show you in simple terms just how easy it is.

I want you do something for me right now, and for yourself. I want you to forget about all of the struggles that you've had in weight loss. I want you to forget about every one of them. Because when you see the truths that I'll show you in this book, and you find out how easy it is, you're going to wonder why you haven't already accomplished it. But at the same time you'll be able to see it. This is not a strange way or road that you have never traveled before. You have traveled this road your whole life.

Diet is the way of life. It is a method or a system in which you have chosen what you would eat or drink all of your life. We've all chosen what we were going to eat or drink all of our lives. So this is a highway that you have traveled all of your life, but maybe you've gone in the wrong direction. You will see how to turn around on this same highway and go in the opposite direction. You will make a U-Turn. It is going to be very easy. It is going to be very natural.

One of the other meanings of the term "way of life" is your path in life, or your course, or your habits of life or conduct, or your eating habits. Seeing that the old path in life (old habits of life and conduct) took you the wrong way, the truth will set you on the right way and this will be of your way of life forever. This way has already been proven to work; it just worked in the wrong way. If you do not believe the system that you have followed all of your life has worked in the wrong way, just look in the mirror. You'll find that it definitely worked. Now you are going to use the identical system that worked for you the wrong way, you're going to turn it around and I'm going to show you how to use it the right way for weight reduction, health and healing.

The word "way" is a route or the road that you choose to accomplish the life you want. What a person usually eats or drinks daily affects them in most every way of life. In the same way, what a person regularly reads and listens to is a diet as well. Look at this: what you regularly read and listen to, what you think about, what you meditate on, what you ponder concerning food and drink, food choices that is what you will do—it will be who you are. That's exactly what Webster's Dictionary says and it's also what God's word says, *For as he thinketh in his heart so [is] he.* [Proverbs 23:7]

Another definition of "way of life" is a course of action or manner of doing something. You want a way to cut back and have the desired weight reduction easily. I will show you through this course of action to have the weight reduction you want. And it will not be hard at all.

I will repeat this many times because I want to instill this inside you. I want to program it on the inside of you. I want to wash your brain with the truth that weight reduction is easy. All of your life you have been told or you've told yourself how hard it is to permanently get rid of weight. Even when you decided to go on a diet, you knew it would be difficult, not even realizing the whole time you were already on a diet—just the wrong kind.

Instead of "going on a diet" why don't you just change the diet you're on? A way of life is a usual or customary manner of living or acting or being. You will learn a different direction, and the different direction will be a way of life. It's not hard; it's easy. I will tell you this over and over again. It's easy. One definition of "way of life" is to have a pleasant way. The truth in this book will show you how to have weight reduction in a pleasant way.

Can you imagine getting rid of all of the excess pounds on your body and doing it in a pleasant way? Can you imagine getting rid of all of them and not being under pressure or strain? Not being under any of the attacks? Not being tormented? Just doing it the right way and not going the wrong way any longer?

Even though they may be somewhat effective, most diet plans try to get you started before you're prepared to start. In other words, you'll see this diet plan and say, "All right, I'm going to go on this diet plan, I'm going to start it. I'm going to start it tomorrow, the next day or I'm going to start it tonight, or whenever." So you'll start this diet plan but you have not mentally prepared yourself to start the diet plan.

The right way to success is to simply turn it around, not put it in reverse. Most diet plans tell you to put it in reverse, or cut down on eating the wrong foods. I want you to understand something. I told you that you were already on the highway that you needed to be on, but that you just need to make a U-turn. You're going to stay on the same highway but you're just going to go in the opposite direction. You're really not going to change anything you're already doing; you're just going to find out how to approach it in a different manner. You're going to see how going the wrong way has given you the problem and the excess weight on our body, and when you turn around, it'll just reverse the process immediately, and it will not be a strain at all.

You're going to go the opposite way on this road, but you're not going to put it in reverse. What I mean by that is simply that your way of eating has been pointed in the wrong direction. It's like if you're going the wrong way and you put your car in reverse. You will be backing up in the right direction, but you can't back down the road forever. You can't just continue to back up and back up back up, because sooner or later, you're going to get tired, or have a wreck. You have to learn how to program your mind to make a U-turn on this highway I've been talking to you about, this way of life, this diet plan.

Instead of "going on a diet" why don't you just change the diet you're on?

Once you know the truths I will share in this book, you won't go the wrong way anymore. You will learn to make a U-turn and totally take your vehicle (your body) that you're traveling in from one point to another, and turn it around and go the opposite direction. That's good, isn't it? And it's not hard to do.

When you're going backwards it's like you're eating wrong and the whole time you're telling yourself, "I'm going to be on this diet, but I hate it. I'm not going to eat certain foods anymore but I still want them." If you're like I was, you're constantly telling yourself, "Don't eat this," but your resistance isn't because you don't like it. Rather, you really do still like these foods, but you've decided that you're not going to eat them.

Let me ask you a question: How long are you going to deprive yourself? How long do you think that you're going to stop eating something if you really really still like it? How long? Think about it for a minute. Let's use some common reasoning with this. Just think about it. How long do you think that you will actually go without something if you really want it? Until you lose five pounds? Until you lose ten pounds? Until you lose twenty pounds?

It's wonderful if you lose ten pounds, even better if you lose twenty. It's wonderful if you lose any amount of weight, but if you don't change your attitude, if you don't change the way you think, if you don't change the way you feel, if you don't learn how to change your taste buds, if you don't learn how to change the way you look and think about different foods, more than likely you'll go back to it.

If you don't believe this, ask yourself how many different diet programs have you been on. I want you to be honest with yourself. If you're like me, you went on hundreds of them, and maybe you were somewhat successful. Let's not say they didn't do any good at all, because they did. Give yourself credit for what you did at that time. But you did not reprogram yourself, change your thinking. You lost some weight and had some success, but you kept thinking the same old way. Anyone who keeps thinking the same way can never expect to get different results. How can you expect to get different results if you keep thinking, acting and talking the same way?

As I said before, you were on the right path for weight loss, but you were simply going about it the wrong way. You were going in the opposite direction, and the key to going in the right direction is not to put it in reverse, but to turn around and head in the right direction. Done the right way, weight loss will not be a constant fight or struggle anymore. Your way of life and diet will be turned around and you totally change directions. The right approach does the right thing. You're going to go the right way of life, you're going to have the right thinking, and seeing as you are doing it the right way, then you will succeed.

You will prosper because you will be prepared before you ever start changing your eating habits. I'm going to show you how to prepare yourself so thoroughly that you will desire to start eating the right foods. You will change it around. If you were going to plant a garden would you just say, "Okay, it's time to start, I'm going to plant my garden" and just throw the seed out there? Or would you get the ground ready first? Which one? You'd get the ground ready and then you could expect good results. After you plowed and broke the ground up and fertilized it, then you would plant your seed. You wouldn't plant it before that; it's the same way with your weight reduction. Adjust your way of eating. Prepare yourself with the words of your mouth and the meditations of your heart. Plow, till, fertilize the ground: your mind, will and emotions; and this will change your direction for you without a struggle. It will totally change it.

This is pretty powerful, isn't it? We've been afraid of the word "diet" all the time and the answer was right in front of us. All we had to do was open up Webster's Dictionary and discover that our fears were unwarranted. Did you know that in regards to the word "diet" Webster's dictionary lines directly up with the word of God? Both of them say the same identical thing.

Let me give you another meaning out of Webster's Dictionary for the term "way of life." It's what one desires. You must create a desire in your heart, in your mind, will and emotions. How can you create a desire in there? One thing you need to know is once you create a desire, God Himself says that you cannot be denied. It is impossible for you to be denied once you create a desire. How can you create a desire? With the words of your mouth, and your thinking and meditation. It will create a desire in your mind, will and emotions and then it will be impossible for you to be denied. The word of God says that God will give you the desires of your heart (Psalm 37:4).

chapter
2
Preparing to Prosper

I want you to apply this first because it is very important. What you do in life always begins with a thought and always involves an internal conversation. Every action in your life was conceived as a thought before it was ever put into action. Some people say, "I wasn't thinking when I did or said that." That's not correct. They were thinking—but just in the wrong way. You cannot do something that you haven't already thought about. Yes, people react on reflex in situations, but these too were conceived with thoughts or "training" over time.

For instance, when you're hungry, you will begin to have a conversation first in your mind, and maybe with someone else, which will lead to the food choices you make. You ask yourself, "Do I want this, or that?" And you make this decision by the habits you have formed. You've formed those habits by how you were taught, which affected your thinking. You may not have realized this, but this is what you did.

You didn't start life eating excess amounts of certain things; you had to be trained. You may have been trained by your parents, or you may have trained yourself. Either way, you were trained and this training often comes by words. Every person is "spoken over" in the sense that words are spoken into their lives with the purpose of having an impact in their lives. You may not have considered this to be truth, but it is. The Bible term "prophesying" is simply speaking into a person's life. People speak into your life every day, whether you or they realize it or not. Words have power and are intended to accomplish something—to either bring death or life. We'll learn more about this later.

Once you were spoken over either by your parents or someone else, then you automatically began to think about those words. When you speak or hear words you automatically think about them. So you're going to begin to revise your thinking simply by talking differently.

Begin to think differently about what you do on a daily basis. You have probably considered why you haven't been able to accomplish weight loss. You've probably tried pills, powders, had operations, and some of you have just tried exercising. There's nothing wrong with exercising. But exercising doesn't have to be the diet plan. It doesn't have to be, I've proven it. I didn't exercise at all and got rid of over one hundred pounds. Should you exercise? Most certainly you should exercise. And you know what else? You don't need a gimmick to get rid of it.

Most people who have struggled with weight loss want the answer. So far, the answer has been to change your eating habits through depriving yourself, a pill or powder, or through exercise, or having an operation. But still this hasn't worked for you. The problem is that these things were done without changing the way you think and talk. While you were looking for the solution in a program, pill, operation, or exercise regimen, the solution was right in the dictionary under the word most people fear the most: diet.

I want to show you something, and I want you to consider this very carefully. Why do they run commercials on TV over and over and over again? Any successful advertising campaign is rooted in repetition. If a person wants his or her product to be successful, they must be willing to make an investment in repeated ads over a period of time. You can't judge the success of an advertisement by what happens in the first day. You can't even judge what's going to happen in the first week. You can't even judge it by what happens in the first month. The media (TV, radio, newspapers, internet) will run an advertisement over and over and over again. Why? Because they have found out that repetition works.

Repetition convinces you to try their product, and they believe that if you try their product you will like it and continue to use it. Because of the effectiveness of repetition, I have heard people tell me things they thought were truth, when in fact, it was really a commercial that had made an impression upon them. They presented it to me as if they had researched it, as though they knew it to be the truth. They were convinced it was the truth because they had heard a commercial over and over and over again.

Isn't it amazing how much television guides our lives? You may wonder what this has to do with a diet plan. I'm going to tell you. What do you see on TV all the time? You see commercials concerning food and drink products because they know that what you hear and think on the most is what you will do. Commercials create a desire in your mind to govern your food choices. The restaurant chain Red Lobster makes appealing commercials because they want you to eat at *their* restaurant—not at another one. They know that when you see their commercial, it will cause you to think and ponder about eating their food because they have made their commercials to create a desire in you.

Advertisers have learned that repetition will work to convince you to try their product and like it. It convinces you because you've heard it over and over again, which causes you to think on it. Then the internal conversation begins and you rehearse it over and over again. It was really a commercial that convinced you of it.

Your diet (what you eat and drink on a regular basis) is driven by what you read, talk and think about day and night. A diet is a system in which you pick and choose certain foods to eat and drink. So as you can see everyone has a diet. Therefore, the word diet is not a bad word or system to be afraid of or shy away from any longer. Instead of shying away from the word diet and the system of a diet plan, you're going to dig into it and find out the truth about it and you're going to win.

Weight reduction will come your way, and I'm going to show you in this book how to have weight reduction, how to accomplish the goal you want—whether you want to lose just 5 or 10 pounds, 100 pounds, or even 500 pounds. Yes, you can get rid of 500 pounds if you need to. It's easy, and you'll accomplish it one pound at a time.

Yes, I used the word "easy." You may have been on many diets before but you've never gone about it the right way. It's all in how you get started. If you don't start in the right direction, you can't end up at the right destination. Let's go back and break it down.

According to one of Webster's Dictionary's definitions of diet, if I change what I read and what I talk about and what I think about certain foods and drinks, I will automatically change what I eat and drink on a regular basis. This will automatically change my way of life. It will change it. I love that word automatically. It automatically changes me. When I change the words that come out of my mouth and the meditations of my mind and heart, I will automatically over a period of time change what I think about certain foods. Yes it will automatically change it.

Automatic refers to lack of struggle or strain. When something is automatic it is not hard.

Notice I didn't say "instantly." When one hears the word "automatic" they usually interpret this to be instantaneous when it's not. Changing the way you think doesn't occur overnight, just like a television commercial isn't designed to impact you overnight, but over time. Automatic isn't necessarily instantly or at once. Automatic refers to lack of struggle or strain. When something is automatic it is not hard.

In the past you went on a diet plan and you struggled with it the whole time, you fought with it the whole time. But you know it's another thing when you can change the way you think about eating and change what you eat and not be restrained and not be tormented. The instructions in this book will teach you how to eat properly and not be tormented. It's one thing to give up your favorite food, which may be chocolate cake or something else and be tormented over it, but it's another thing altogether to give it up and not be restrained over it or tormented at all. You just turn around and walk away from it.

> *Whatever you read, talk about, and think on day and night will be prosperous in your life.*

I want to go back to the word automatic. My car is an automatic, and when it's running good, all I have to do is put it in gear and start down the highway in the right direction. Do you remember I told you earlier that the term "way of life" is part of the meaning of the word diet? The way of life is the road you choose to travel. We do that every day in life; we get in our cars, put it in drive and start down a certain road or highway.

Why do we choose a certain road to go on? Because we have a certain destination or point where we want to arrive, and usually we want to get there in the quickest amount of time. Do you see what I'm saying? Therefore, we choose that road; we choose our way of life.

What you're going to do is to choose a road to go down to meet your destination point which is a proper amount of health and reduction in weight. You're going to reduce your weight and you're going to have fun doing it, and that's the truth. You're going to go down the highway in the right direction. When I'm going down the road in the right direction I'm motoring along, I'm in automatic. I don't have to change gears; my car automatically changes gears for me when I get to the right speeds. Did you notice that in automatic there's no strain, no struggle for me to change gears, it just automatically changes gears?

Again in automatic there's no struggle. When I'm doing it right, as long as I keep the car serviced it will automatically change gears. You have to check and service your vehicle or your way of thinking on a regular basis. You have to check and service your way of talking on a regular basis too.

I said this before that referring to the word "diet" Webster's Dictionary lines right up with the word of God. What I read and what I think about, I do. Joshua 1:8 says that what you read, talk and think on, you will do. *This book of the law shall not depart out of thy mouth; but thou shalt meditate therein day and night, that thou mayest observe to do according to all that is written therein: for then thou shalt make thy way prosperous, and then thou shalt have good success.*

This is not just a book for reading only, but one of participation. In order for this to work for you, you have to participate in what I'm sharing with you. If you wanted to build up muscles in your body and exercise then you would have to participate in the right way of exercising. If you want to accomplish something at work you have to get started in the right direction and you have to put action to it. Your way of life will be according to what you read and talk about on a regular basis.

The Bible says when you put action to your words, thoughts, and meditations, then you shall make your way prosperous and you shall have good success. Whatever you read day and night, whatever you talk about day and night, whatever you think on and ponder day and night, you shall do (Joshua 1:8).

I want you to notice the word "shall." The word "shall" is the most absolute word in the English dictionary. By simply changing your words and thinking that you must change them forever then you will do it. You will do those things that you read, talk about and think on. Whatever you read, talk about, and think on day and night, will manifest and be prosperous in your life. You're going to bring prosperity into your life concerning weight loss.

This means that you will do it, that you will accomplish it, and that you have a new way of eating for health and weight reduction.

What does it means to prosper? Jesus said that you shall be justified by the words of your mouth (Matthew 12:37). Isn't that amazing? The word "justify" means to be rendered free. Now if you're free, you're totally unrestrained, or not under any pressure or temptation. When you're free, you're not tempted to eat the wrong foods. Jesus said that the words of your mouth will cause you to be free. Jesus also said that the words of your mouth will also cause you to be condemned; or in other words, cause you to be bound or stay in the same old situation in life.

It's not wise of us to think we can continue to do the same old thing and get different results. If I'm going to get different results then I've got to approach it in a different way. Think about how many diets have you been on. It isn't good to think about all your past failures but I want you to consider how the other diets have not worked for you. Why would you continue to do the same thing and expect different results? What I'm sharing with you in this book is different, so you should get different results. If you follow what I teach in this book and do it the right way, you will accomplish your goal this time.

To prosper means that you will develop hope, you will develop a goal, and you will develop a vision. Did you know that the word of God says that when you do not have a vision you will perish? (Proverbs 29:18) By proper conversation and proper meditation concerning the right food choices you will be able to get a vision and develop a dream in your heart to eat the right things. It's that simple. You will develop a vision of health, of proper weight reduction.

To prosper also means to flourish, and succeed with speed. If you follow the simple instructions in this book, you will not only succeed, but you will succeed with great speed and great success.

Weight will come off your body quickly when you approach it the right way. It's just like when you get in your car and go down the right road to get to the right destination point. If you go the wrong way and if you don't adjust it, you won't reach your destination point. But if you approach it the right way and go down the right road then you will get there quickly.

You might ask, "How quickly can I get there?" This depends greatly upon how much weight you need to get rid of. I got rid of over 100 pounds in nine months. That's excellent, but do you know what's better than that? I kept it off! That's the key. The key is not to just get rid of it, but to keep it off. You've probably lost some weight before, but then you went back to your old way of living and gained it all back, and maybe even more. By the method in this book, I got rid of over 100 pounds and kept it off.

To prosper means that you will get it done quickly and forever. When you follow the Godly principles which are in this book you cannot fail. Weight reduction will come quickly and easily. It says that you will thrive, that you will grow in accomplishing your goal and that it will happen in a vigorous way. The words of your mouth and the meditations of your heart convince and cause you to line up your life with spiritual principles. The word of God is filled with spiritual principles. The diet of words and thinking directly affect what you eat and drink.

I didn't have a doctor tell me this, nor do I claim to be a medical doctor, but I do claim to have gotten rid of over 100 pounds. I do claim to be in excellent physical condition. I will tell you that I have excellent blood pressure. I'm telling you that every time I get a physical they give me a clean bill of health. I'm telling you that I'm healed and I'm not sick. I'm telling you that I'm not excessively over weight anymore. I'm not saying that being overweight is bad, but it's bad for your health. You don't want to be overweight and you know it and it bothers you. And I'm telling you that you can get rid of excess weight if you'll change the words of your mouth and the meditations of your heart. I didn't learn this from a medical doctor. I learned it through the word of God and I learned it by practical experience. If you will change the words of your mouth, you will change what you eat and drink and you'll actually change your taste buds. You'll change what foods you desire to eat and drink on a daily basis.

Prosper also means "to be," which means you have arrived, you're there. You're not just trying to make it, not just struggling, but you have arrived. When you prosper you have special insight. Did you know that once you get insight on something you cannot be stopped from reaching your goal or purpose? Once you get revelation, once you get enlightenment you cannot be stopped—it's impossible. God created you to be able to accomplish anything good in your life. God created you that way and all you have to do is to get insight into it. God created you with an inner ability to get insight and the way you get insight is by talking it, thinking it, meditating on it, and pondering it day and night, over and over again. Once you get insight on it then you cannot be stopped from accomplishing it.

Since prosper means to be, this means that you are no longer trying to be, you are no longer trying to accomplish weight reduction because it means that "you are." You are now doing it. To be means "I am."

Prosper also means to accomplish. This is wonderful! This is awesome! The words of your mouth and the meditations of your heart will cause you to do it. And when you start doing it, you've automatically moved into it without strain or struggle. I started doing this before I started the different diet, the change of diet. The whole time I was getting rid of over 100 pounds, I started changing my thinking process. Once I accomplished changing my words and thoughts, accomplishing the diet was as easy as walking through my house or getting into my car and putting it in drive and driving somewhere.

It is not hard to accomplish weight reduction if you start on the right road first. To prosper means to accomplish. Now get this: saying it, thinking it, talking about it day and night causes you to do it, and when you do it, this causes you to prosper and behave intelligently. Isn't that amazing? You can behave intelligently concerning food and drink choices automatically. You will no longer allow wrong words to come out of your mouth.

To prosper means that you will learn to consider before you act. It means that you will behave intelligently. You can go to a restaurant and look at the menu and make good choices. You won't have to say, "Oh, I just slipped up today." You'll make good choices concerning food because of your words and thoughts. However, if you do mess up, don't worry about it; get right back in there and get started and don't quit. You will win if you don't give up.

Did you know that God designed you to be a winner? When Jesus said that you will not perish but have everlasting life (John 3:16) part of the meaning of the word perish means that you will no longer lose. If you're a born again Christian, you have the God given ability to win every single time, to never lose again. Jesus said that you will not perish.

Part of the word perish means you will not be destroyed, you will not be marred, you will not be scarred and you will no longer lose. You don't have to lose anymore. And not only did He say that you don't have to lose, but He also said that He has given you the power to make right choices. It's right on the inside of you. And when you speak proper words and give proper meditation and thoughts to those words, then you will make the right decision.

Prosper also means to be an expert. You will be able to instruct others how to do it. You're not just accomplishing weight reduction and proper health, but you will reach the point where you can instruct others also. Isn't that wonderful? Not only can you get rid of excess weight on your body, but you can also instruct others how to get rid of the excess weight on their body.

Prosper also means to be prudent, skillful, and able to accomplish. This is wonderful. When you prosper you make wise decisions. So not only are you winning, you will have the wisdom to get rid of the excess weight—weight that did not belong to you anyway.

I will never gain it back; and I mean never. I want you to think of this and conceive it deep down in your heart. Excess weight does not belong to you. It is an intruder. You need to look at excess weight as an intruder to your body. If someone broke into your house, that person would be an intruder. You would do everything in your power to get rid of him. Now you have the power to run this intruder off, to get rid of this intruder off your body. Who in the world would want a small thing like food to control their life?

Think about it. In the past I allowed a piece of cake or a candy bar to control my life. I told you in my testimony that I had a habit of eating six or seven sweets a day, not including the sweet sodas I was drinking every day. It's a total shame that I would allow that to control my life. It doesn't control my life anymore, but I allowed it to control me. Your body belongs to you and you need to start taking authority over it. You need to start telling your body what it will eat and what it will not eat. You need to start taking authority over your body all the time. Take authority over it.

Remember that excess weight on your body is an intruder and you are going to make it leave. It doesn't have a choice. You control your body, you own it. Your body belongs to you, and you're going to make this intruder get out of your body. You're going to make this intruder leave and it's going to leave forever. If it ever tries to come back you're going to say no.

When we're prospering we have help on the road of getting rid of excess weight. Remember that Webster's said that diet is a way of life. You're going to succeed in reaching the goal and have a prosperous journey.

The word prosper means to be happy and well off. I'm on a

special diet program. There are certain foods I do not eat any more. I've changed it and I'm happy about it. I doubt you've ever been on a diet before that you were happy about it. But with this method, you're going to be happy about it.

Not only have you won and have gotten rid of and are continuing to get rid of excess weight so it will never return, you're also happy. You'll be at peace all the way through it. That's what reading this book will accomplish for you. You will not be tormented at all; you'll be totally free and unrestrained.

Because prosper means to accomplish, it also means to fulfill completely, to execute, to terminate the problem, and terminate bad food choices. You will terminate them and extinguish them for life. You will do it. You're not going to start on a weight loss program and get part of the way through it and quit. You're going to finish the course. You're going to win.

To prosper means to me to" make perfect," to perform and even go beyond. In other words if your goal was to get rid of 100 pounds then because you're prospering, you're going to get rid of 102 or 103 pounds. You're going to go beyond, to finish it. It's your goal and your vision together to get rid of x number of pounds and you're going to accomplish that plus go five pounds over. The effects of this spiritual law go exceedingly and abundantly beyond what you can ask or think. God's word says that you will have good success.

Having Good Success

Let's talk about what it means to have success or succeed. Prospering makes the way for you to succeed. God said, *You shall make your way prosperous and you shall have good success.* You will make your way prosperous by choosing to say the right things, by choosing to meditate and think on the right things, then it will cause you to automatically do the right things concerning weight reduction and health. It will cause you to automatically do the right thing, and make your way prosperous. The Bible says that you shall make your way prosperous and then you shall have good success. It says that you have developed your hopes and your goals and your visions. It says that you will prosper in weight reduction and flourish with speed, that you will get there quickly. You will be able to follow it without any trouble. Weight reduction will be quick and easy.

You will make it happen through the word of God, through speaking it properly and meditating on it properly. You will become an expert at it, and you shall have great success. You will cause yourself to be well off, to never return back to the old things and you shall have great success.

Do you know what else? Not only will you accomplish weight loss, but you will do it in a safe manner. To be successful means that you are doing it in a safe manner. You will do it with no fear, dread or torment. Most of the time you dreaded every other diet you went on before you got started. This time you're not even going to dread it. Because you will change your words and thoughts, you will move into it automatically and it's not going to be a problem. Weight reduction will no longer be associated with fear, dread and torment but associated with pushing forward and coming out mightily, causing you to be profitable. This causes you to be prosperous, and you'll always take the right path, which means that you will arrive in the shortest time period.

Success comes from the mouth and from the heart, and from the meditations of your mind. This spiritual law will work for you. It will take an active part on your behalf to begin it. You will open your mouth and speak the truth. You will say the right things about yourself from this day forward. It will cause you to be careful and consider the right thing and relate it to circumstances. You will get rid of this weight and it will not be any problem whatsoever.

Let's go back to the word "diet." I want to go back over it with you because I want you to see it. I want you to know that it's the truth.

The word diet refers to a meaningful influence, a way of life. A diet is a regimen; it's what a person usually eats or drinks on a daily basis. A diet is also what a person regularly reads and listens to, or a special or limited selection of food and drink chosen and prescribed for weight loss and for health. Both are intended to accomplish something. It is going to happen for you and it's not going to be any problem whatsoever. It is very simple. You take the words of your mouth and the meditations of your heart you begin to change what you say over it. Let me give you an example.

I'm going to make it so simple that you cannot miss it. If you like chocolate cake, you just simply begin to tell yourself that you do not like chocolate cake anymore. I know that sounds foolish and maybe crazy, but the way to good success is done by learning to call things that be not as though they are. You change things around by the words of your mouth. You take the thing that be not and call them as if they were. The "be not" in this case is your dis- like of chocolate cake because in the natural

Why would you continue to do the same thing and yet expect different results?

you like it. But if you say, "I don't like chocolate cake anymore," you're calling the thing that is not as though it is. Doing this will change your like of chocolate cake into a dislike of chocolate cake.

Right now you need to simply make a vow to yourself. The vow you're going to make is not that you're not going to eat a certain thing anymore. But rather, you're going to vow that you will never eat foods that are bad for you again without first talking to yourself and speaking to that food or problem in your life.

I'll use the example of chocolate cake again. You will never eat chocolate cake without first talking to it and telling it, "I do not like you anymore I will never eat you again and I don't like the taste of you." For a while you'll turn around and eat it anyway, but that doesn't matter because you didn't make a vow to never eat it again. Your vow was to never eat it again without first talking to it.

Every time you think about chocolate cake, you tell yourself how much you do not like it, how much you don't like the taste of it and that you're never going to eat it again. Think about what you're telling yourself, ponder on it. You may say, "I feel like I'm lying."

You're not lying—you're following God's example by calling things that be not as though they were. What you're doing is changing your mind concerning this piece of food. This is what you're doing. Then at the same time, you take the foods that you do not like now and are good for you, like broccoli, and you look at them and tell yourself how much you like them, how much you love them, how much you love the taste and that you're going to eat them on a regular basis from now on. It's that simple. You just have to do it over and over again.

chapter
3
Five Steps to Success

Your manifestation is only a very simple five-step process away. Most of you who are reading this book have already gone through at least one, if not two, of these phases. So you would only have two or three more to go. As I explain them, you will see how simple they really are to understand or accomplish.

Now remember there are five steps in the process of manifestation. You already have the power and ability on the inside of you to accomplish this, but these five steps will lead you to the manifestation of your weight loss. I'm going to call each of these five steps an arena.

1. "I don't want to"
2. "I want to"
3. "I can"
4. "I will"
5. "I am"

Arena 1: "I don't want to"

The arena where most people begin is the arena of "I don't want to." Many people say, "I do not want to go on a certain kind of diet; I do not want to change the way I live." Actually they want to get rid of the excess body weight, but they are just thinking that. However, they don't want to change their eating habits. Doing it the way I teach in this book and finding out the truth, you'll find out that if you just simply change your thinking, then you will change your eating habits. It is very simple, and it is very easy.

All you have to do to come out of the arena of "I don't want to" is to begin to change your confidence or persuasion level that's on the inside of you. All you have to do is to begin is to talk to yourself and listen to others who will motivate you. Always remember this, you can hear someone else tell you 10,000 times that you can do it, and you may believe them to a point, but you will never believe anyone more than yourself. That's why you have to continuously tell yourself that you do not like this or that kind of food anymore. All you have to do to come out of the arena of "I don't want to", is repeatedly tell yourself. Even though you don't feel like it, continue to tell yourself, "I want to go on this type of an eating plan so that I can get rid of the excess weight on my body." Then you will come out of the first arena and have accomplished 20% of your goal. You will come out of the first arena and move into the second arena of "I want to."

Arena 2: "I want to"

"I want to" is a wonderfully powerful arena. Now understand this, here's where most people mess up on changing their eating habits or diet plan. They come to the arena of "I want to" and they start the diet plan while they are in the arena of "I want to". Well that's okay, but if you stay in the arena of "I want to" and you never go to the arena of "I can" or the arena of "I will" or the arena of "I am", it is likely that you will go back to your wrong eating habits and gain the weight back. The different arenas develop a tremendous heart's desire to accomplish this mission of getting rid of your excess weight loss and good health. As I go through this you will see what arena you are in. You probably have gone through a few of these arenas with other diet plans but you have never gone to the final arena of "I am" where you will accomplish getting rid of all of the excess weight from your body. Using the principles in this book, I went from a size 50 pant to a size 36, and from a size 3X shirt to a normal medium or large shirt.

I want you to understand that the arena of "I want to" is a fleshly arena; and when you endeavor to "lose" weight, you're accomplishing it by the arm of the flesh. You can achieve a certain amount by the arm of the flesh. You may lose a pound; you may lose ten; you may lose thirty or even fifty pounds; but the problem with just losing weight and not "getting rid of it" is that most of the time you end up re-finding what you have lost. You don't want to do that. You don't want to look at this as a "weight loss program." You want to look at this as a weight reduction program, a way of getting rid of it permanently. I'm going to say that again, "getting rid of," not just losing but getting rid of, that comes from changing your lifestyle. Excess weight does not belong to you. It is an intruder. Don't forget that, it's an intruder.

What is the meaning of "I want to?" You saw diet plans before and you said, "*I want to* go on that diet plan; *I want to* lose this weight." Listen to this, the word "want" means to have too little of. In other words, you can't have a *want* if you don't have a need. You're basing your *want* on your need, and you can't just stop at your need. The word of God in Philippians 4:19 says, *My God shall supply all my needs,* but you know it never says He's going to supply it according to the need. It says that He'll supply it *according to his riches and glory by Christ Jesus* or through the strength of God Himself. So when you get to the arena of "I want to" you are recognizing that you have a need. You are recognizing that you have a lack and maybe even a lack of will power, a lack of strength, a lack of ability and that's why you are in the arena of "I want to".

Can you see this? The arena of "I want to" is a good arena to go through. Did you notice I said, "Go through?" In other words, you don't begin the arena of "I want to" and start the new diet plan and new way of thinking, talking, eating, and living, and stay in that arena for the rest of your life. In the arena of "I want to" you're always desiring those foods that you're not eating, you're always wanting them, you're always desiring them, you're always craving them, but you're just depriving yourself with the arm of the flesh and you're forcing

> *Excess weight on your body does not belong to you. It is an intruder.*

yourself not to eat it. You will accomplish this through studying— not just reading, but through reading and studying and meditating on the truths in this book, you will reach the goal when you can say, "I do not want it anymore." When you get to the point of "I do not want it anymore" it's not hard not to eat it. How do you like that?

So you see the arena of "I want to" is a good arena, but it's not the arena in which to stay. You begin with "I want to" and the next arena that you're going to have to go to is "I can." You're climbing a ladder. You have gone through the arena of "I don't want to", where you said, "I'm tired of it; I'm not going to go on another diet; I've tried it before and it didn't work." Now you've moved through the arena of "I don't want to" to "I want to" and once you're through "I want to" then you can move to the third arena of "I can."

Arena 3: "I can"

The arena of "I can" is a more powerful arena. It is not your final destination point but you are half way to accomplishing your goal. The Bible says, *I can do all things through Christ Jesus who strengthens me.* [Philippians 4:13] "I can" means that you have the necessary resolve, the courage to reach your goal of getting rid of excess weight. You're not just wishing or hoping; you're not just a longing for it, but now you've arrived at the point where you have the courage to accomplish this mission.

"I can" means you are able to do it. It means that you are able to accomplish it, if you only would. It means that you are able mentally to do it. Do you hear that? It means that you are able mentally to do it. I love that. Being able mentally means that you are moving out of the flesh of "I want to" and you are beginning to move into the spirit realm and you're beginning to reach the point of "knowing." When you reach the point of "knowing" then you've come a long way. "To know" means to perceive, comprehend, to understand and have a full working knowledge. When you begin to reach the point of "I know" then you'll know that you are arriving at your final destination. You're at the point now that you can begin to get rid of this excess weight on your body and it's not bothering you as much to not eat those certain kinds of foods. Now remember I laid down sweets and I haven't eaten one for two and a half years—not one at all, and it doesn't bother me any way whatsoever.

When you move into the arena of "I can" you're likely to accomplish your goal. This is a good arena to be in, but understand that like the arena of "I want to" you don't remain in the arena of "I can." You say, "I can do it. I can do it this time. I can get rid of this excess weight that does not belong to me anyway that is an intruder." You now have the moral, mental and legal right to accomplish it. You're bringing forth the power out of your inner man to manifest getting rid of all the excess weight that is on your body.

See the word "can" as being a container full of power, ability, and know how. "Can" is a container. It means that you're full of the strength and ability. It means you have the power to accomplish your goal. Don't forget that. You've moved into the arena of "I can" and you have the full power to accomplish it.

Did you know the word of God said that *death and life is in the power of your tongue?* [Proverbs 18:21] In other words, you can condemn and sentence yourself, and you can hold yourself in bondage with the words that come out of your mouth. That's what you've done when you went on those other diets plans before. While trying to deny your flesh, you told yourself how much you liked this food or that food. Let me tell you this, you will only deny your flesh for a certain length of time. The only way to change your flesh is to put it under subjection to the words of your mouth. You can change your taste buds with the words of your mouth. You can cause yourself to not want it any more; you can control your five senses so that they will not control you. You must begin to call things that are not as though they already are. When you look in the mirror, tell yourself, "I do not like this food any more." In doing this, you're washing your mind, you're washing your brain, you're washing your will, you're washing your emotions. You're cleansing yourself, and once you get yourself clean of the wrong kind of thinking about the wrong kind of foods, then you will be able to control your five senses. Yes, things may still smell good, but you'll say, "I don't like that anymore." And the more you tell yourself that you don't like it anymore, the more you will change your taste buds and line yourself up to the proper way of eating.

It's not hard when you line up your mouth and thinking. When you line up your mouth and thinking, you've aligned your heart and your mind, will and emotions and instead of you serving them, they will serve you. That's exactly what's going to happen. You'll look at excess weight as an intruder. If someone broke into your house, you would do everything possible to get them out of your house so they couldn't steal from you. The excess weight on your body is stealing your health—it's destroying you and going to put you in your grave early. You don't have to put up with it, and you've already reached a place of "I can" get rid of it. Because excess weight is an intruder, you will do whatever is necessary to get rid of it. You'll get rid of it one pound at a time, one ounce at a time.

If you don't think one pound is much, get a stick of butter out of the refrigerator and you'll see how much one pound is. One pound or even five pounds is a lot of weight and you need to rejoice every single time you get rid of an ounce. One pound is not your final destination, but it's better to only have to get rid of ninety-nine more pounds than it is a hundred. Rejoice with every pound you get rid of and give thanks to God every time. Rejoicing will give you encouragement; it strengthens you

See the word "can" as being a container full of power, ability, and know how.

and it moves you on down the way. You begin to put a spiritual force into action that works for you and not against you.

After you get started, it doesn't matter that you didn't get rid of any excess weight. That's not the issue. The issue is a change of lifestyle. If you move into the fifth arena of a change of lifestyle ("I am") then you will have accomplished your goal and it will manifest in your body.

But on the other hand, when you complain, it puts in motion a spiritual force that works against you. Do not complain. Do not murmur. It keeps you from achieving; it affects you in your mind, will and emotions, and you will not feel like continuing. But if you encourage yourself, you will make it. You need encouragement. Being glad and rejoicing is in your favor, so do it. No matter whether you feel like it or not, do it, and you will accomplish every single time.

Now that you've moved from the arena of "I want to" to the arena of "I can," say this to yourself, *I can do all things through Christ Jesus who strengthens me.* I do have the strength, I do have the power, and I do have the ability. Look in the mirror and tell yourself "I can get rid of this excess weight that is on my body." Remember this—the arena of "I can" is not the final arena, but now you are more than half way there; you are 60% toward your goal of full manifestation and of changing your entire life.

Arena 4: "I will"

The next arena that you're going to move to is a very powerful arena and that is the arena of "I will." In the previous arena, you acknowledged your power to get rid of the excess weight. Now your words will be, "I will accomplish getting rid of the excess weight that's on my body."

In the arena of "I will" you have the three "Ds", which mean you have Decided, and you have begun to Declare it, and you're going to Decree it. You're going to decree, "I will." You're no longer saying, "I can do it." You're now saying, "I will do it". There's a big difference between "I can" and "I will" as the former describes ability, but the latter conveys a willingness that comes from this power.

When you say, "I will" you're making a choice or decision. You're at the stage of making choices and decisions. You are now at the point where you are controlling your own actions. You're not just responding to a desire for candy or ice cream. You are now making those desires by choice and you're creating the right desires in your mind. You are now controlling your own actions instead of your actions controlling you.

When you move into the arena of "I will" you have not reached your final destination point, but you're now strong; you're not weak any more. You've moved past "I can" into the arena of "I will" get rid of the excess weight on my body. You're fixed, you now have a purpose, and you now have that vision, and like a plant with deep roots, your goal is deeply ingrained in you. Your goal not going to be uprooted easily. A little bit of a discouragement is not going to get you to quit now. You'll overcome a little bit of discouragement with determination. Where there is a will, there is way, and you will accomplish this new way of life.

When you move into the area of "I will", it creates energy and enthusiasm. In the arena of "I will" you don't get tired as easily; you're full of strength, courage, and enthusiasm. It also affects your disposition and your attitude towards the matter. Now you're happy to make the choices. When you move into this arena and you become happy to make the right choices. You are now arriving. You are now almost at your final destination point and you're happy. Being happy is a byproduct of joy, which is a spiritual fruit that comes from the inner man. In the arena of "I will" you are now producing godly fruit. You will not be denied, you're 80% toward changing your life.

When you move into the arena of "I will" you are now developing proper desires. You're not going by the old desires anymore; you're not making the wrong food choices anymore. You're making the right food choices as a byproduct of the right desires. When your desires begin to change, your taste buds begin to change. I'm telling you that I actually changed the taste buds in my mouth. A lot of people don't understand that, but once you get a hold of this one truth, and begin to apply it to your life, then you will see for yourself.

When you move into the arena of "I will," it creates a compelling demand. I demand my mind to think properly and to make the right food choices. I demand my will to line up with right food choices, and therefore I'm choosing willfully to make right food choices instead of wrong ones. I put a demand on my body to obey me. When before they used to lead me to making wrong food choices, I now put a demand on my five senses to help me make right food choices. I decree it. I put a stamp *You are now controlling your actions instead of your actions controlling you.* on it. In the Old Testament when a king put his ring on it he sealed it, he put a stamp on it and it was law, and it could not be changed unless he superseded it with a higher law.

Once you've moved into the arena of "I will" you will accomplish your goal. This is a power where you actually will yourself into action and accomplish it. You will yourself into the area of success. You now have developed the power of choice and you have a deliberate action resulting from this power. You're creating the desire in your heart, in your mind, will and emotions, and once you have this desire you cannot be stopped. Did you know that once you've created a desire in your heart, a real deep-rooted desire (not a wish, not a hope so) you cannot be denied? It is totally impossible that you will be denied.

You have a right to be the right size and not have the excess weight on your body. Because the right sized belongs to you, you demand or call for it in an urgent way. You have a right to be free because Jesus said that the words of your mouth will cause you to be free and totally unrestrained. He also said that the wrong words coming out of your mouth will condemn you or hold you in bondage (Matthew 12:37). Making wrong food choices and having excess weight being on your body is bondage and you will get rid of it. You are getting to the point where you're demanding your appetite to obey you and to line up and do what's right.

Now remember that you've moved from "I don't want to" to "I want to". Then you've moved from "I can" to "I will" where you are making demands on your mind, will and emotions. I can guarantee you when you continue to make those demands, you will control it. Then you're not wishing, you're not hoping. You know. You're demanding that your taste buds line up, and you're in control. In the arena of "I will" you now begin to tell your body and appetite what it will do and what it will not do, instead of the way it used to be. You will change your habits; you will change your taste buds. Minute by minute they will change. Hour by hour they will change. Day by day they will change. Month by month they will change. They will change forever because you will change.

Arena 5: "I am"

Praise God you have now arrived! You're in the fifth and final arena called "I am." Say this, "I am what God says I am." In the arena of

"I am" you're eating properly; you're eating healthy; and you're eating what you're supposed to eat. You're not even worried about it anymore. When you've reached the point of "I am" you're not wishing, hoping, not even praying for it to come to pass. You've already got the answer. It's here. It's manifested. You now see yourself as having arrived. Once you get to this point then you will have revelation knowledge of the truth in this book, and once you get enlightened knowledge of the truth of this book then you cannot be denied. You'll be able to see; you will not stumble; you will not fall. You will not make wrong food choices one day and the right food choices the next day. You'll live the rest of your life this way and it will not be hard and you'll do it now because you want to. Even your "want to" will line up, your "I can" will line up, your "I will" will line up because of "I am."

When you've reached the fifth arena, you're not trying to make it happen anymore. It's happening now. You're no longer getting there, you're not arriving, but you *have arrived*. You have won. You are the winner. This will happen to you long before you get rid of the excess weight on your body. You reach the point of "I am" before even starting a diet plan.

I reached the point of "I am" before I ever started eating properly. You can reach the point of "I am" a third of the way of getting rid of all your excess weight, a fifth of the way, or half way. The key is not when you reach the point of "I am" but the key is reaching the point of "I am." In your spirit, you are already in the realm of "I am" but you must get your soul (mind, will, and emotions) to realize it.

Then you are fully confident; you are fully persuaded. You look in the mirror and you see excess weight on your body but you're not persuaded by the flesh, you're not persuaded by your natural ability anymore. You are now fully persuaded that you have accomplished your final destination. You've got that spiritual force behind and you cannot be denied. You cannot be turned down. Most of the time this happens before you ever get all of the excess weight off of you. It can also happen before you get any of it off but your manifestation will arrive. Every bit of it will come off at this point. You have now created a deep-rooted hearts desire and you cannot be stopped. It is impossible, you cannot be stopped, nobody can stop you, no group of foods, no new foods, no power can stop you, nothing can stop you now.

Let me tell you what it means to have a deep-rooted desire. It's a desire of your heart. It's now your companion, your process. You now resemble that deep-rooted desire. When you have that desire it means that you have reached completeness—full maturity. You have moved into what is called perfection. You have now become one with your heart's desire. You have created a oneness, a singleness. You are now single-minded towards the goal or the vision. You're not double-minded anymore.

According to James 1:7-8, when you're double-minded, you're not able to receive anything from God. It doesn't say that you can't start down the path, but it says that you can't receive full manifestation when you're double minded. When you reach the point of "I am" you have reached the point of single-mindedness. You're focused upon your goal, your vision. You now have that vision before you, a vision you will

> *When you've reached the point of "I am" you're not wishing, hoping, not even praying for it to come to pass. You've already got the answer.*

fully accomplish. You will not be denied, you are not worried if you can make it, you're not wondering if you can make it, but you are now single-minded. You are focused towards that final destination point of getting rid of all of that excess weight off of your body. You will make it. You cannot be denied. It is impossible now for you to lose and all you have to do is to continue to renew your mind to the right way of eating and you will make it.

In the fifth arena "I am," you have created that deep-rooted heart's desire. You are now one with this desire and you cannot be stopped. You have reached the point of completeness, of full maturity and you will not be denied. Praise God you have now arrived. You will now reach your full manifestation of getting rid of all of the excess weight that is on your body that is an intruder and it does not belong to you anyway. Remember to stay focused, stay single minded. Every time a wrong thought comes in, you say "no, I will not think that way concerning that food I am not supposed to eat. "

Yes, you should talk to yourself. Remind yourself of the truth and do not be held in bondage to wrong foods any longer. You have now accomplished and you will get rid of the excess weight that is on your body.

Remember that all of these arenas are good except for the first one, "I don't want to." The second one "I want to" is a good arena, but remember it's a good arena to go through, not stay in. The next arena "I can" is a great arena. You've now reached the half way point; don't forget it. "I can" is also a great arena to be in, but you have to go through it, and move to the fourth arena that decides, declares, and decrees, "I will." That's a good arena but you have to go through it in order to get to the fifth arena of "I am" and the divine influence of God will be behind you. The numeral 5 stands for grace throughout the word of God and the divine influence of God will help you. It will move in your heart and you are now persuaded that you are the winner.

Once you accomplish these five arenas in your life, then you will not go back, because you will continually be renewing your mind in the proper manner and cleanse your mind in the proper way. You will be doing that from the arena of "I am" and the arena of "I am" means that you have fully accomplished the mission and you will see it.

chapter

4

<u>Know the Truth and Be Free</u>

I want you to forget the past. Do not ever again rehearse your failures in weight loss. Forget all the times you have tried and failed. Forget them. Get rid of them right now, and know that you approached the other methods the wrong way. It wasn't really your fault because you were just not properly educated or informed. Once you know the truth, it is not hard to accomplish getting rid of excess weight on your body. It is not hard whatsoever. It is very easy and very simple.

Most people say that in order to lose weight you must close your mouth. But I tell you to open your mouth; open it wide and open it often. Begin the right way. Make a vow right now that you will not eat another wrong food unless you first talk to yourself. You need to tell yourself how much you do not like it, how much you do not like the taste of it and the fact that you will never eat it again. Will you eat it again in the beginning? Most likely you will. Most likely you will eat it again in the beginning but you must talk to yourself over and over. Then you will be able to reach the point of knowing the truth.

Jesus said, *and you shall know the truth and the truth shall make you free.* [John 8:32] Now I want point out something to you so you can see this with me. It's only the *truth that you know* that makes you free. Jesus said, "You." He made it personal, and makes it like the word "whosoever." That's what you've got to understand. It brings it down to whosoever.

Whosoever knows the truth, then the truth that they know is

what makes them free. Freedom is not hard to accomplish. All you have to do is bring truth on the scene, and truth will automatically make you free. *You shall know the truth and the truth shall make you free.* Being as truth automatically brings freedom, and I said automatically – you see something that's automatic is simple, it is easy. Being as truth automatically brings freedom, undoubtedly we have not known the truth about weight loss and getting rid of excess weight off of our bodies or we would have already accomplished it.

> *It's only the truth that you know that makes you free.*

Getting rid of excess weight is not difficult. If you were like me, most likely you have always thought that weight loss was difficult, that it was almost impossible if it weren't actually impossible. At one time in my life I was totally convinced that I did not have the power or ability to get rid of all of the excess weight that was on my body. I weighed 300 pounds believing that I would have to live that way the rest of my life.

I will prove to you that it is easy to get rid of excess weight on your body and that anyone (or whosoever) can do it. It's the same for one person as it is for another. If you're not watchful you'll read this book and listen to my testimony in the beginning of this book and you'll say, "Wow, that's wonderful for you but that doesn't fit me."

You've got to understand when Jesus said, *and you shall know the truth and the truth shall make you free,* that you are a whosoever, and once you know the truth, it will manifest freedom. As I said earlier, weight loss is automatic when you bring truth on the scene. I'm not talking about just losing ten or a hundred pounds and gaining it back because you went back to the same way of thinking and consequently, the same eating habits. I'm talking about getting rid of it forever, and I mean forever. Can you see that?

I want you to begin in your mind to form an image of yourself at a smaller weight—with the excess weight off your body. You begin to now create a picture of yourself that is not overweight and you get it fixed firmly in your mind and keep it there. Now you're going to accomplish this forever.

There are three very important things that we need to know. You shall know the truth and the truth that you know shall make you free. It shall cause you to be totally free. And let me emphasize the word "shall." Earlier, I mentioned how the word "you" is a personal word. The word "shall" is a word that is used in the Greek to explain an absolute. In other words, there is no other word that explains an absolute more than shall. Shall is such an absolute that God is telling you that if this were not already created, then He would create it just to meet your need. That's how strong the word shall is. Shall is totally absolute.

You shall know the truth and the truth shall make you free. I want you to notice that this does not say, "You shall know the truth and take three pills a day and you'll be free." This does not say, "You shall know the truth and you'll mix a powder with it and be free." This does not say any of that. Furthermore, this does not say that you'll know the truth and go through an operation and be free. I'm not criticizing you if you have attempted any of these methods to get rid of excess weight. However, if you don't change the way you think, even though you may have an operation, you're likely to gain that weight back if you're not careful. The word of God also does not say, "You shall know the truth and exercise and lose weight." Exercise is good and profitable, but exercise isn't required to get rid of excess weight off your body. Without changing your thinking, you'll have a tendency to have to fight it all the time.

You can still have a refrigerator in your house. Open the refrigerator and if you know the truth, you'll still be free. It says that you can go out to restaurants and still eat properly and be free. We are talking about a change of life. We are talking about a change that is forever, one where you will never go back to being the wrong way.

Know the truth and be free. Remember that weight loss is easy. What's easy is not hard, nor is it difficult. In the past, and I know – I've been there, it's always been hard, it's always been difficult, you've always had a struggle even though you lost ten or twenty or however many pounds it was. I started on diets in the past and didn't even make it the whole day. I have been on them and have lost some weight, but I always gained it back because I didn't do it the proper way.

You need to know this, excess weight on your body does not belong to you. It is not yours and you do not ever refer to it as being yours again, never, ever. Don't refer to that excess weight as yours. It is not yours; it does not belong to you. Consider excess weight as an intruder. An intruder doesn't have the right to be there and it's not going to stay there. You used to think that it belonged to you, but now it's going to leave. It will never come back once you know the truth about how the way you talk and think as it relates to the way you eat and drink.

What is Truth?

Know the truth and be free. You must find out what truth means. I've learned that when I explain truth to most people, they don't even know what truth means. They don't understand truth; they don't know what it means. They think truth is just a bunch of facts compiled together. That is absolutely not so. From this study, you're going to find out what truth is. Truth automatically brings freedom. If you don't have freedom in any area of your life, including excess weight, then you do not know the truth yet. Truth has not arrived. Excess weight cannot stay on your body when truth arrives concerning right food choices. Truth is absolute. There can be no exceptions to truth. It is impossible for a mistake to be in truth. Listen to this, truth has absolutely no change in it whatsoever. What was truth yesterday, what was truth last year, what was truth in 1950, what was truth in 1800, what was truth when time actually began as man knows it, what was truth then is still truth today. Truth cannot change. Truth will never change. Truth is the same yesterday, truth will be the same today, truth will be the same tomorrow, and truth will be the same throughout all eternity.

Truth is pure—it has no mixture. Truth has no mixture of partial facts whatsoever. There again, just because it's fact does not mean that it's truth. It cannot be truth if it's partial. You can compile numbers of facts together but they still may not be truth because truth is absolute.

I once viewed a TV news report where they admitted they had lied to obtain facts, which caused certain people and organizatons trouble. Those facts, no matter how many of them were accurate, could not be compiled into truth. Yes, some of the facts were accurate, but the whole story was not truth. Very seldom do we ever hear a truth because normally we hear facts and then we hear someone else's opinion concerning the matter. They say it's not their opinion, but that's not true.

This is truth: Jesus said in Matthew 12 that your words will cause you to be free. When Jesus said that your words will cause you to be free or your words will

> *Once truth is brought on the scene, you will have full light. You will know where you're going.*

cause you to be sentenced and condemned and held in bondage then He meant it. The word of God says that life and death, freedom and bondage are in the power of the tongue. This is truth, and by no means can it be changed. Truth isn't truth just because I believe it to be truth. It doesn't mean just because you believe it or you agree with it that it's truth. Now you have to believe it before truth can set you free, but truth itself automatically brings freedom—once you know it. It cannot be partial truth; it must be 100% pure to be truth. Remember this, according to Jesus Christ Himself, the words you speak cause you to be free, and they also cause you to be held in bondage.

You do not have to help truth. Truth will automatically cause you to be free—it's an absolute freedom. Truth, when it is applied to your life, automatically causes you to be free. Truth is a reality. It is vibrant. It is powerful. Truth always has the power to cause or to bring freedom. You cannot deny truth once truth is brought on the scene. Once you know and perceive truth then you will automatically be free. You will not be held in bondage to making wrong food choices or having excess weight on your body.

Truth is a certainty. You are now certain, you're stable. Truth means to be stable, to be fixed, and it means to be without doubt. How do you like that? Once you bring truth on the scene you will never have anymore doubt whether you will accomplish getting rid of the excess weight.

Truth is light. There is no darkness in truth. Since truth is light, no darkness can remain around truth because light chases away darkness. Once truth is brought on the scene you have full light. You will know where you're going. You will know how to arrive. You will not have any fear. You will not have any doubt. You will not even wander off course, because you can see the light and you can see the way to travel now.

Since truth is certainty, and all doubt is out, you're now operating in faith. You are convinced that all of this excess weight will come off your body and you're not even worried about it. You'll know that you have arrived. Truth is loyal. Truth will never forsake you. Truth is accurate in all its descriptions. Truth causes you to have devotion. Truth causes you to always accomplish your goal. Remember, there will be no more struggle in it. There are no more wrong decisions in truth. When truth arrives, you'll never make another wrong decision; there's always a surplus. Did you hear that? There's more than enough power. There's more than enough of strength for you to make right food choices and cause this excess weight to come off your body. I like that. It has equity. It's more than enough to cause you to be an overcomer. You're more than a conqueror once truth comes on the scene.

Truth again is the same yesterday, today and forever. It is unchangeable. It doesn't matter what your opinion is. It doesn't matter what my opinion is. It doesn't matter what the opinion of some scholar is. Truth cannot be changed. Truth is something that is fixed. It is firmly placed and attached. It is unmovable. Truth is established. Truth is settled. Can you see how truth automatically will cause somebody to be free?

Once truth comes on the scene you're firmly making right food choices without a struggle, without a strain. It is unmovable. It is attached. It is established. It is settled. It will remain in the same position and you don't even have to make it stay there. Truth automatically stays in the same position. Truth will cause you to control your thoughts and actions. Truth is like a covenant. It is a binding solemn agreement.

Jesus said the words of your mouth will cause you to be free, will cause you to overcome, and will cause you to arrive. By you telling yourself that you do not like these wrong food choices anymore, this will cause you to arrive. You tell yourself you don't like them, you tell yourself you don't want them, you tell yourself you don't like the taste of them anymore. The words of your mouth will cause you to arrive because the words of your mouth will bring life and health to you, and they will cause you to get rid of this excess weight off your body.

The words of your mouth will change your mind. You don't even have to try and change it. All you have to do is speak the words, even if you don't believe them in the beginning. Speak them, think about them, and do it day and night and after a period of time you'll begin to believe them. Once you begin to believe them, you'll begin to act on them, to follow them. You'll begin to do them and the excess weight will come off your body and you will be prosperous and succeed beyond a shadow of a doubt.

Truth is like a powerful formal contract that cannot be broken. Did you see that? Truth is like a powerful formal contract that cannot be broken because God established it. It is impossible for truth not to work. You can't move truth out of the way once it arrives on the scene. All you have to do is apply it, and you'll be free. You have to learn what truth is. As I said earlier, most people don't understand truth but you will. You will understand truth. I'm going to tell you what truth is from every angle. It's important that you know what truth is. You have to know truth and it's only the amount of truth that you know that causes you to be free. But if you don't know what truth is, you will never know it. How are you going to know, perceive, comprehend, understand, have a full workable knowledge and be able to apply it to your life and show others how to apply it to their lives if you don't even know for sure what it is? You have to know what truth is before you can apply it.

Once you've learned the meaning of truth, then you can learn what it means "to know" and then you can be free. You'll also learn the meaning of freedom. As I said earlier, truth doesn't have any doubt in it. Not even the devil himself can stop truth from working. It cannot be stopped in any way. Truth will build you up. Truth will support you. Truth is power to you, causes you to never be weak. It causes you to never come to an end. Truth causes you to never fail. Where truth is, it is impossible for you to fail because it is impossible for truth to fail. It is impossible to come short of the goal of weight reduction, of getting rid of this excess weight off of your body.

Truth is stable. Truth is not easily moved. Truth is never thrown off course. Truth is firm. Truth is steady. Truth will not break. Truth is trustworthy, you can depend on it. It is reliable. It is worthy of your trust. Truth is stable and it is firm in character. When you know the truth it causes you to be firm in character and in purpose. It causes you to be firm in your goal in your vision. It causes you to be unchanged. It causes you to know that if you need to get rid of 100 pounds that you will accomplish it. You will know that you are in that position. You will feel different. You will feel good about it. You'll feel good every time you lose one pound. You'll rejoice over each pound. Truth is reliable. Truth is unchangeable. Knowing the truth causes you to be mentally sound. It causes you to have sound foundation. Truth automatically changes your mind, will and emotions, all you have to do is apply it to accomplish your goal.

As I said earlier, facts can change. You have to understand this. History books tell us that at one time they thought the world was flat. This "fact" was based on the knowledge they had at that time, and it was a fact in that day according to man's knowledge. But let me tell you, truth is unchangeable. The world was round then and the world is still round today. There were stars in the sky then and there are still stars in the sky now. There was a sun and a moon then and there's a sun and a moon now. It is totally unchangeable. Truth is the same yesterday, today and forever.

Truth causes you to be sure. It will cause you to speak with full confidence. It will cause you to make certain decisions. It will cause you to be confident in your decisions. It will cause you to be sure of yourself. It will cause you to have solemn confidence. It will cause you to have an inward guarantee that all of that excess weight will come off of your body, that you shall arrive at your goal and you shall not be denied. Truth causes you to have good eating habits and choose the right foods. You will not choose the wrong way anymore. You will only choose the right way. You will no longer be defeated. You will no longer struggle. You will now set up a new way of life. Truth causes you to have a new way of life permanently and forever.

You will be able to prove it. You'll be able to demonstrate it. You'll end up building a good reputation. You'll be able to win and make right food choices. It brings to you security or a state of feeling secure. Truth brings freedom and certainty. It assures safety and protection, a defense against attacks. When you start having wrong thoughts that come to your mind, all you have to do is bring the truth forward and it's an automatic protection against wrong thinking.

Wrong thinking brings wrong results. Right thinking brings right results. It causes you to escape wrong thinking. Truth will guard and protect your new lifestyle against all invaders. It will do it every single time. When you know the truth you shall be free. Then you become confident; doubt and fear are defeated – don't forget that. Unbelief leaves. Doubt and fear cannot stay in the same place where truth is. It is impossible. No two substances can occupy the same place at the same time. When truth arrives it automatically casts out doubt, fear, and unbelief. Therefore, you are automatically confident in what you're doing. You're not held back any longer. You do not doubt any longer. Doubt, fear, and unbelief are your worst enemies and truth expels those things. How could you not win? How could you not succeed? It's impossible for you to not win. Getting rid of excess weight off of your body is not hard—it's easy. You cannot lose when truth arrives.

Truth is the state or quality of being free. That is an awesome truth. Truth is the state of being independent from making wrong food choices. With truth, you're independent from doing the wrong thing. You're free from the influence and control of wrong food choices. What foods influence you now will not influence you then. What seems to have control over you now, will not have control over you then. Truth is the most powerful force in the universe because truth is developed from God Himself.

"To Know"

What does "to know" mean? Know is a powerful word. It is wonderful when you know something. Most people do not know, they think they know. Remember the scripture – you shall <u>know</u> the <u>truth</u> and you shall be free. I just got through telling you how absolute truth is. We learned what truth is and when we find out what "know" is, then we will automatically be free. I'll also show you what being free means. Most people don't know what it is to be free.

To know means to apprehend or to understand. I'll give you seven definitions of what it means to know. Seven always stands for completion or completeness:

1. to know or have knowledge of
2. to perceive
3. to comprehend
4. to understand
5. to have a full workable knowledge
6. to apply it to one's life
7. to teach others how to apply knowledge to their lives

When you know the truth of a certain matter, then you can apply it to your life. If you are not able to apply it to your life then you do not <u>know</u> it to its fullest extent.

To know means to know it, to perceive it, to comprehend it, and it means to understand it. You can comprehend it; you can take it in. Did you get that? You can take it in. You can comprehend it. You can understand it. It means you have a full workable knowledge of it. In other words, you don't just know it on paper, you don't just know it because a book told you, you know it in your "knower" on the inside of you. Your mind knows it, your will knows it, and your emotions know it. Everything gets involved in knowing. You are able to apply it to your life and you're able to show others how to apply it to their lives.

I want to show you something very important about the word "know." To know means to apprehend. In other words, if you know the truth then you can now apprehend it. You can understand it. You can take hold of this truth, to never again let it go. You have a full enlightenment of this truth. This results in being the right size and getting rid of all excess weight on your body. Can you see how the truth of this book will cause you to accomplish getting rid of all the excess weight off your body and how that it's really not hard? Can you now see why you haven't had success in this before?

It's not difficult to understand. It's not hard to apply to your life. All you have to do is open your mouth the right way, think about it the right way, and you'll automatically begin to do it. You'll automatically begin to prosper and you'll automatically become successful. It's not hard. This is simple. A ten-year-old can apply it to their life. Let me tell you something, you've applied it all of your life even though you didn't know it. You just didn't apply it the right way. Once you know this truth, you will never let it go again, resulting in being the right size and getting rid of all the excess weight off your body. You will now take the truth into custody; you will <u>know</u> it. You will capture it concerning getting rid of excess weight. You have now taken hold of it mentally. It is now affecting your mind. It is now affecting your will. It is now affecting your emotions.

"To know" means that you have a clear perception of it. As you can now see clearly, it will never be hard to see the right way again. Never. Being as you can see clearly, and as you can understand, you can now perceive how to get rid of death and choose life; how to get rid of bondage and choose freedom. Accomplishment is in the power of your tongue. Can you see that? Nourishment is in the power of your tongue. Ability is in the power of your tongue. Recovery is in the power of your tongue. Becoming alive the right way is in the power of your tongue. You will love it. You will love the results of this new life.

You will say, "This is good. This is a good life. This has brought me freedom. This has refreshed me. This has made my life strong. This has caused me to have a pleasant life and not be tormented. I have perceived this. I have learned this. It is good, efficient and beneficial. It is restoring me to health and soundness."

Proper words affect your whole spirit, mind, will, emotions and body. Therefore, they affect your life. Knowing has caused you to be firm, to have a mental grasp of the truth. When you know the truth, it is firmly planted in you. It's like the method of grafting one plant into another plant or one fruit into another fruit. That's what you're doing with these words of your mouth, you are injecting them into the realm of your thinking. You're injecting them into your mind, will, and emotions. You're engrafting them into you. Once it is engrafted into you, it becomes an integral part of you. You don't have to just try to make it happen, and try to say the right thing, and try to make the right choices. You will now automatically make the right choices.

The truth is now firmly planted into me because I have engrafted it into me. I now have it securely in my memory bank. That's part of what knowing is—you know it, it's securely in your memory bank and it will never come out. It will never be deleted. The only way I can take it out is to take it out on purpose, and I will never take it out.

If you know something or someone, it means that you're acquainted or familiar with it. You're intimate with it. It's a part of you. It is actually a pleasurable experience of yours. Excess weight is being removed from your body and it's easy, not a struggle. You have understanding, which means that you now have the skill to apply this newfound truth to your life. You will open your mouth and speak these truths. You do not like the bad foods and you like the good foods. You recognize and distinguish right from wrong. Once you know it, you are able to distinguish right from wrong in the manner of all food choices.

The issue is how much to eat. You will be filled and satisfied with the right amount of food. You don't have to go back for seconds all the time. Because they are now conformed to the image that you have planted in them, your mind and emotions will obey you. You will do this when you know it: know, perceive, comprehend, understand, have a full workable

I saw myself the right size before I ever lost over 100 pounds. I began to know it, to perceive it...

knowledge, able to apply it to your life, and able to teach others to apply it to their lives.

You have now created an image of this on the inside. God has given you the ability to create images. The creation of images is not bad. It's just what images you create that can become bad or be good. In my case, I had the image of myself being overweight. I had the image of eating wrong foods. I had the image of eating five or more sweets a day and drinking six or seven sodas a day. I had an image of overeating all the time. That's the kind of image I had on the inside of me.

But by the words of my mouth and the meditations of my heart, my mind, will and emotions, I now have a new image of me. I don't see myself as being fat anymore. I see myself slender. I see myself the right size. I saw myself the right size before I ever lost over 100 pounds. I began to know it. I began to perceive it, and comprehend it and understand it. I began to have a full workable knowledge of it.

I'm not making myself out to be something I'm not. But I'm telling you that you have the power to create images on the inside of yourself. Our mind is like a computer, and all we have to do is program it. We will erase what we don't want in the computer anymore. The old life is no longer a part of me. I don't have to fight and struggle over wrong food choices.

Every once and a while a wrong thought comes to me. I'm to the point I don't even have to resist that thought anymore. Because I know the truth, I just laugh at it, because I know that thought is not a part of me. I know that thought does not line up with the image I've created on the inside of me. I've said it so many times and I still say that I created a new image on the inside of me and that new image is not fat. The new image does not have all kinds of excess weight on it. The new image is more slender. The new image is in better health. The new image follows what it's supposed to follow.

Once you create a new image on the inside of you, it's not hard. Once you see yourself that way, all you'll do is follow what you see. If you can't see it, you can't have it. Part of the meaning of the word know is to see (perceive). You can see it now. Once you know it to the fullest extent, you can see it. Don't criticize or condemn yourself over being overweight; just do something about it. Start saying the right things. Start having the right meditations. Start having the right thoughts. You can control your thoughts with the words of your mouth. Once you say it so many times you'll automatically begin to think it, good or bad. This is an absolute and it cannot be changed. You will have a firm mental grasp; don't forget the truth is firmly planted in you.

Don't forget you are grafted by knowing truth. You have engrafted this truth into your mind, will and emotions. This truth is now a part of you. Isn't that awesome? It's now a part of you, you're acquainted with it, you are familiar with it, you actually experience it, you have understanding of it, and you now have skill to apply this newfound truth and open your mouth and speak it out and enjoy it, and love to eat the right foods. It's actually a pleasure for me to eat the right foods. Why? Because that's what I want now. The wrong foods don't matter any more; they are not an issue. How much to eat is not an issue because I know how much to eat. And the whole time I'm doing it, I'm enjoying it because I'm going by the truth. I have full confidence. I don't have to stay away from certain restaurants.

My wife will say, "Honey, where would you like to eat tonight?"

And my answer will be "It doesn't matter, honey. Wherever you wan to eat."

It doesn't matter if we go to the Chinese place, I'm going to eat right. It doesn't matter if I'm going to eat Italian food, I'm going to eat right. It doesn't matter if I go to the steak house, I'm going to eat right. I know what's proper on my diet, and I stick by it. I don't go in and act like I'm scared; I'm going to eat. I know the truth, it's now a part of me, and it's engrafted in me. As I said before, when you engraft one plant into another, the new plant reproduces what was always true of both of those plants together. The portion of one plant that you grafted into the other plant is always with that plant when it reproduces from that time forward.

You're getting rid of your stinking thinking. You're now in the arena of "believing." Your mouth is a weapon. It is the front edge of a weapon. This is something you need to know. Your mouth is the front edge of a weapon, and you have to use it <u>for</u> yourself and not against yourself. Every time you say the right thing, those words begin to be joined to you. Words are containers. They are containers that are full of the elements that make up the word. If I'm speaking right food choices, I'm dumping what's in that container in me. I'm bringing myself to health.

Here's the meaning of the word mouth: it means gash in the face, opening in the earth, but it also means front edge as of a weapon. Your mouth is a weapon. If you don't believe it, get into an argument with someone and if you're not watchful you'll use your mouth as a weapon against that person. Your mouth is a weapon and you need to use that weapon against wrong food choices. You use it against wrong food choices and then you take your mouth and you use it as a weapon in your defense for right food choices. It is your choice how you do it. Don't forget the meaning of the word mouth: the front edge as of a weapon.

I want you to know this also that the word of God says, "*As a man thinks, so is he.*" [Proverbs 23:7] It says that because it's truth. You shall know the truth and the truth shall make you free. Let's look at the word "think." Do you know what it means in the Greek? It means to open. So as a man thinks in his heart, his mind, will, and emotions, so is he. So then, whatever a person opens himself to is what he becomes—how he acts, and what he does. That's as simple as you can get. It's not difficult to understand. When you tell yourself how much you love those right food choices, you're opening up your mind, will and emotions for the good stuff to be poured in. In the past, you opened your mind, will and emotions to the wrong thing to be poured in. Now, don't allow the wrong thing to be poured in anymore. Allow the right things to be poured in. Put your trust in what the word of God says. "To think" means to open yourself to it, and it says what you think about will affect your mind, will, and emotions. That's the way it works.

> *Words are containers. They are containers that are full of the elements that make up the word.*

Once you know the truth you cannot be held back any longer. You cannot be defeated. It is impossible for you to lose. You will reach your goal. It doesn't take the truth and a pill; it doesn't take the truth and a powder; it doesn't take the truth and an operation; it doesn't take the truth and some kind of gimmick; it doesn't take the truth and some exercise; it doesn't take the truth and anything else—just know the truth.

The power and ability is in you to accomplish anything. All you have to do is know the truth. That's all you have to do. It's not hard. It's not difficult. To know means "to know, to perceive, to comprehend, and to understand." You will know the truth and you will be free. You shall accomplish and get rid of all of the excess weight that is on your body. You have the ability and the understanding.

Truth is security in your mental bank. Did you hear that? Truth is security in the mental bank and it's actually a part of your being once you add it like I'm telling you. Once the truth is secured in your mind, the truth will never leave. It is a spiritual principle, and you take the words of your mouth and you engraft it into your mind, will and emotions, and you cannot lose. It is totally impossible for you to lose because when you *know* the truth, you have a clear perception of it.

Knowing it means to know, perceive, comprehend, understand and have a full workable knowledge of it, being able to apply it to yourself and also able to apply it to others. Yes, that is the way it operates. It does change your life and it will change your life forever.

Being Free

I want you to know what it means to be free. You probably never felt free when you went on a diet before. You always felt a pull on you, a nagging, a compulsion to eat the wrong foods. The reason for this is because almost every diet involves restraint of some kind. When you feel restrained you're not truly free.

When you begin to understand freedom, you'll be unrestrained. You're able to accomplish it. You're not only able to get rid of the excess weight, but you are able to do it with pleasure. Imagine getting rid of excess weight and doing it with pleasure. Being free means that you can now be exempt from torment, that you're not obligated to the wrong things anymore. These foods no longer control you.

I am totally unrestrained. Thank God almighty, I am free. The truth has made me free. It has brought me into liberty. It has brought me to where I absolutely make the right food choices with pleasure.

Once you realize the truth that *you have*, and not the truth that someone else has, you will have the power to denounce wrong foods and put them under your feet forever. You are on the road of freedom that has no restraints. You are no longer a slave to wrong food choices. They do not control you anymore, but you have charge over them and you control them. Free means that you are not re-strained any longer—you are exempt. Did you get that? You are now exempt. If you are exempt from something it has no more part of you.

I am now exempt from wrong food choices. I have total lib-erty. I am now free to go into any restaurant and it does not bother me. I'm free from wrong food choices. Because I'm free, I'm not worried; I'm not tormented; I'm not even compelled. Because I'm free, I'm not even tempted anymore.

Did you know that being tempted means you are hard pressed to doing something? If you're exempt from it, how can you be tempted? Think about it. You say, "Oh everybody is tempted." No, you're only tempted when you're drawn away by the lust of the flesh. You can only be tempted in those areas where it is possible for you to submit to it.

In my case, I'm not tempted to eat sugar any more. Eating sugar is not a temptation to me. I'm exempt. I'm free. I'm totally unrestrained. Freedom causes me to break through. It affects my integrity and my reputation. Once I'm free, I'll build a reputation on it. This freedom equips me. It cleanses me. There's no more guilt in me. When you're overweight like that you have guilt in you. There's no more guilt in me. It as if I was never guilty.

My mind has been cleansed. It's like I've never been that old person, but only the new person. *As a man thinks in his heart so is he.* Don't forget it. Like a gatekeeper, you have to be watchful over the words of your mouth and over your mind. Like a drawbridge of an old castle, you draw the bridge down to allow in the right thoughts, to allow in the right words. If it's wrong you draw the bridge up, you do not let it in. You do not let yourself think of wrong food choices, only the right food ones. You are now totally free.

Remember that words dictate your thinking and as a man thinks so is he. Words are containers, and you will deliver the right things to your mind, will and emotions, which will deliver it to your five senses. It will deliver it to your taste buds and they will be changed. Don't think of yourself as unprivileged; don't think of yourself as deprived to where you can't eat this or that or the other anymore. Don't feel that way. Remember to say this… "I can. I will. I am. I have accomplished the goal. I am accomplishing it all the time. I am getting rid of all the excess weight that is on my body and I'm enjoying life praise God. I'm telling others about it. I'm helping others. I not only have a hold of it, but I'm helping others."

> *Free means that you are not restrained any longer — you are exempt.*

To be free means that you are totally free. You have now been rendered free and you will not be bound anymore. You are not restrained any longer and you are now totally free.

chapter
5

Free

We have been discussing the word of God that says, "You shall know the truth and the truth that you know shall make you free." It is an absolute that once you know truth and apply it properly, then it will make you free. I want to continue with this thought about knowing truth and being free and what it means to be free. It is very important that we understand what freedom is all about.

When you are free it means that you are not under the control of the wrong food or food choices any more. Did you get that? When you're free, you are totally unrestrained. In other words, if wrong eating still torments you and holds you in bondage, then you are not free. You must understand that. If you are not free yet, there are only two reasons. Either you do not understand and know truth, or you are not applying that truth by knowing it completely. Because when you really know truth you can apply it to your life and it will manifest. Therefore, to be free means that you are not under the control of wrong foods anymore. You don't have to be so concerned with getting excess weight off of your body as you do with making right food choices. Once you learn how to make right food choices then you will automatically get rid of excess weight from your body.

When you're free from something, it no longer has any power over you. Most people who haven't had a problem with wrong eating habits would not look at food as having power over them. But anything that dominates your life has power over you, instead of you having power over it. You must understand this. It doesn't matter whether it's food or something else—it's the same thing. Food and wrong food choices become addictions for people, just like alcohol, drugs, and many other things in life. They become addictions to you, and you become addicted to eating wrong foods, just like I was addicted to eating sweets.

I've mentioned a number of times in this book that I was addicted to sweets, eating as many as seven sweets a day not counting the sweet sodas. But it's worth repeating. A lot of folks are not addicted to six or seven a day, but addicted to three or four a day. Or they may be addicted to other wrong food choices and it's the same thing. But when you're free they do not have any power over you anymore in your actions or your thoughts.

If you believe you can't control your thoughts, you are wrong because you can. You can definitely control your thoughts. Every thought that comes into your mind you can bring it into captivity (2 Corinthians 10:5). All you have to do is take the proper words and speak them on a constant basis, and you will take into captivity the thought that's telling you to eat the wrong foods. You will take that thought into captivity and end up casting it out of your mind and replacing it with correct food thoughts. I can go into any restaurant and still eat the right foods. It's one thing to eat the right foods in restaurants but it's

When you are free it means that you are not under the control of the wrong food or food choices any more.

another thing when you can go in and not even desire to eat the wrong foods. That's a whole different ball game. That's freedom. That's what happens when you get free.

Once you know the truth and you move into freedom, you don't want to eat the wrong foods anymore. You don't desire them anymore, and you very seldom ever think about them. And if a thought flashes through your mind, you just cast it out. It won't be a problem for you. When you're free, you are not restrained. I've seen people go on a diet and say, "Well I'm not going to eat any of that chocolate cake but I sure do want it."

I've got news for you. The chances are that if you want it bad enough, sooner or later you're going to start eating it again. It's the same way with an alcoholic. He can resist for only so long while still having the desire to drink. But if he associates with people who are drinking, and this desire still has power over him, more than likely he'll begin drinking again.

Everyone can be free. Being free means that it does not have any power over you anymore in your actions or thoughts. There are no restraints. Once you're free you have total liberty to eat in any restaurant you want to, and you don't have to be afraid. I've heard other people say,

> *Once you're free, you're at the point where old food choices are totally uprooted out of your life...*

"No I don't want to go eat in that restaurant; they're serving food I'm not supposed to eat and I want to stay away from it." This way of thinking is restrictive and just as much bondage. When you're free and your desires have changed, there will be no restrictions. I don't expose myself to things that are harmful, but let me just say this to you. If I'm with my family or a group of people and they want to eat at a restaurant and they ask, "Where do you want to eat?" I say, "It doesn't really matter to me" because I know that I'm going to make the right food choices.

It does not matter to me. I don't care. It doesn't bother me. I'm telling you what it means when you move into freedom. And if you're not to this place concerning wrong food choices then you're not yet free. But always remember this: once you know the truth you shall be free, once you know it. For you to know anything, it has to become a part of you. I don't know if they still teach this, but when I went to school they taught us multiplication tables by memorizing them. I sat down and I told myself over and over and over that 2 x 2 is 4, or 10 x 10 is 100, or 5 x 8 is 40. I told myself over and over and over until I had it in my memory bank; and now that I have it in my memory bank I can recall it any time I want.

What I did was to tell myself that I didn't like certain foods. I would stand before the mirror and renew my mind to what I already knew. You have to continue to renew your mind to what you already know. You don't want these truths to fade. Don't allow them to be washed away; renew yourself to them. I used to tell myself probably as much as fifty or a hundred times a day how much I did not like certain foods and how much I liked other foods. I would tell myself constantly and intentionally. I want you to notice this: I intentionally reprogrammed myself, because I found truth from the word of God. Renewing your mind by the word of God is how you reprogram yourself and get yourself in the right order.

I have no fear of going into any restaurant with anyone and eating the wrong foods because wrong foods are not in my vocabulary; they are not in my memory bank; and they are no longer a part of me. Once you get free, you're at the point where old food choices are totally uprooted out of your life and cast away from you, and the right food choices take their place. Once that happens, it's as though poor food choices never were. Hallelujah! Now that's what I call being free. That's what I call being free, without being tormented. That's free. It's so wonderful you can apply this to anything.

It's altogether different when you don't even desire unhealthy food anymore. When before you made wrong food choices, now you actually want healthy foods. Being totally free means you are totally independent of it, that you have liberty. You're not under its control. Because I'm free, I'm not under the control of sweets and cake and ice cream and candy anymore. I don't eat it at Christmas. I don't eat it at Thanksgiving. Someone said, "I don't want to be that way." And I said, "Well go on and stay in bondage."

If you're going to be free, be free. You're not looking for relief; you're looking for freedom. Relief says, "I need to get rid of fifty pounds but if I just get rid of fifteen pounds, that's okay. Fifteen's great. Fifteen's wonderful, but fifteen is not fifty. Real freedom brings you into fifty. Do you see what I'm saying? Freedom is not satisfied with partial bondage. I was eating seven sweets a day. Freedom is not satisfied with cutting down to three sweets a day. Because you know what's going to happen? All you're doing is satisfying your flesh and before you know it you'll be right back to seven. That's just the way it works. You've got to uproot it. You've got to get it out completely or otherwise, you'll fall back in. Once you get it out completely, then you're not down to three or four, you're down to zero, and it doesn't bother you.

They can bake a cake in my house and it doesn't bother me when they sit down to eat cake. I've seen other people who went on diets and *lost* some weight, but some of them *found* it again. Their diets would torment them the whole time even if they saw cake. That's not the way it's supposed to be. That's not the case when you're free. When you're totally independent, you're free. You have liberty, you are free. And when you know, perceive, comprehend, understand, have a full workable knowledge and can apply it to yourself and show it to others so they can apply it to themselves, when you know the truth you shall be free.

However, it's only the truth *that you know* that brings you freedom. You're able to move in any direction. You're not held in chains any longer. You're not confined. You're loosed. You're not burdened. You don't feel an obligation to a certain kind of diet. It becomes a way of life instead of an obligation. You're not confined by any patterns or wrong choices anymore. You're not constrained. When you're free, it becomes easy.

How many of you know that you can do anything when it's easy? You can do anything if it's easy. Jesus provided a way of knowing truth so that it would be easy. It's easy to turn and walk away from wrong food choices when you know the truth. It's easy. You become graceful with it. When you become graceful with it, it's not hard anymore. You're generously empowered. You become more than an overcomer. Therefore, you're not just struggling through the day eating the right foods but you've become more than an overcomer. At the end of the day you're still feeling good.

Did you know that once you become free, you're happy to make the right food choices? You're excited about making the right food choices. You see, it's easy to get excited over the results when you see the results. But what about before you see the results? Once you know the truth and you move into freedom, then you become happy making the right food choices. That's what I call being more than an overcomer. When you're free you have an abundance of power. Like I said, it's not just enough to barely make it through the day but more than enough to be unrestricted or unrestrained.

Let me give you another definition of what it means to be free. Being free means you will now be clear of obstacles that are in your way. There are all kinds of obstacles in your way. This is a real world we live in. We're not talking about moving and living inside of a bubble or fantasy world. We're talking about living in a real world of getting up and going to work, stopping at restaurants, eating at home, or wherever you may eat, you still make right food choices. When you're free, it removes the obstacles out of your way. What would be an obstacle or a stumbling block is no longer a stumbling block to you because you choose not to have it. That's freedom. You're free. The road ahead is free. It is clear and without restriction. You're not fastened in any way, you're free. You're set free from any sort of restrictions and restraints and entanglement.

When you say the proper words about the proper food choices and think about how much you like the right food choices, and you tell yourself how much you do not like the taste of the wrong food choices, that becomes a confession to you. Here's what happens: when you first begin saying it, you won't even believe it yourself. You're not just going to wake up tomorrow and say it one time and be free. It doesn't work that way. You've got to purpose this on the inside of you; you've got to continue to say it until you believe it. You must do this.

The objective is to line up the words of your mouth with the believing of your mind, will and emotions of your heart. That's the objective. Once you've lined up your mouth and get your thinking aligned with it and then you'll begin to believe what you're saying. You do not believe anyone as much as you believe yourself. I can tell you all day long that you have the power to overcome—to get rid of this excess weight off your body. I can tell you all day long, but you will not believe it until you begin to tell yourself. When you begin to tell yourself, then it begins to register in your mind. It begins to register in the realm of your soul. Your mind believes what your mouth tells it, and not only that, but your whole body will believe what your mind tells it. That's right. It doesn't have a choice in the matter.

When you begin to confess it, you'll begin to believe it, which means that you are assenting to what you're saying. And when you assent to it, you accept it. When you begin to tell yourself how much you like certain foods that are good for you and you begin to tell yourself that you do not like certain foods that are not good for you, you will not believe it at first. However, after a period of time you'll begin to assent to it, which means you will begin to believe it and accept it. Once you accept it, then your body will begin to accept it also.

Freedom overcomes temptation. What does it mean to be tempted? Being tempted means to be hard pressed. It's like you're pressured and you're between a rock and a hard place. You feel forced when you're tempted. Once you reach the point of knowing the truth and you become free, you're not even tempted any more. You may have a vague thought run through your mind, but it's not a temptation because you're not hard pressed to do it anymore, you're free. You are now agreeing with the words of your mouth. You are consenting to them. You're making a covenant with yourself to eat the right foods and not eat the wrong foods.

As I told you earlier, you don't have to be concerned about the excess weight coming off your body. It will automatically come off if you make right choices. It's not hard at all. You're coming into agreement with yourself. After a period of time you will begin to admit this to yourself. It's like you're promising yourself over a period of time. You don't have to say, "I promise myself that I will eat this all the time and I will not eat this." You automatically promise yourself after a period of time because you are coming into covenant with yourself concerning the matter of excess weight coming off your body and making right food choices.

It's like bringing yourself into oneness with right food choices. You and right food choices are now one. You and right food choices are no longer two different things. Right food choices actually become a literal part of you. That's being free.

We're talking about a law of the spirit realm and laws of the spirit realm cannot be changed or broken. When it's a law of the spirit, it has to work every single time exactly like it's set up to work. Now we have a natural law where the speed limit is 55 and you might get pulled over for doing 65, but you might get out of it. Do you understand what I'm saying? This kind of law is not like a law of the spirit. At the same time, the law of the spirit says that what you sow, you will reap. There is absolutely no way out of it. What you sow, you will reap.

> *Once you reach the point of knowing the truth and you become free, you're not even tempted any more.*

When you sow right food choices you will reap excess weight

coming off your body. You don't have to make it happen, it'll just happen. When you sow wrong food choices, we know what will happen there, don't we? We don't even have to discuss that. We know from past experiences that this is true. You see, it's a law of the spirit, whatsoever a man sows, that shall he reap (Galatians 6:7).

More About Being Free

I want to discuss a little bit more about what it means to be free. To be free means to be liberated. It means to be set free. It means to be released. When you're free, you're released from the slavery of wrong food choices. Once you're free, you are exempt. It means you are no longer obligated. You're no longer held in bondage. You are excused to go free. It's like getting out of prison. Making wrong food choices is like being in a prison, and it seems like it's hard to get out. But it's not hard to get out if you do it by the law of the spirit and begin to speak and meditate day and night over and over. Doing this will automatically lead you to freedom.

To be free is to be delivered. You're not held in bondage any longer when you're free. This symbolizes that you have carried the wrong food choices to a faraway place and left them there. You have uprooted the wrong way of thinking and replaced it with right food choices. When you're free, you do it with pleasure. If you have not reached the point of eating the right foods with pleasure and enjoying it, then you're not yet free.

Keep working on it. You're not a slave. You're not bound by it. It's like the struggle of getting rid of excess weight is gone, and it came at absolutely no cost to you. It was free. Freedom actually moves into graciousness, kindness and favor. Through the power of the Holy Spirit and by knowing the truth, you now have a divine influence operating in your life that is your assistant. You are continually fed with power and strength that you need to continue on.

Once you're free your choices are spontaneous. Your right food choices become natural in accordance to how you have trained yourself. You are now free. You are no longer tempted with wrong food choices; you're only making right food choices. You're voluntarily doing it without a struggle. You're clean just like a drug addict gets clean. You're now clean from wrong food choices. And it becomes as though it never was and it is removed out of the way. You're exempt from the bondage and you have no more guilt. You're totally innocent, you're clear now, you're no longer guilty, you're dismissed, you're blameless, desolate of it. You're free, you're guiltless, and holy in spirit, soul and body. I'm talking about real freedom. Thank God Almighty, I'm free.

chapter
6
Whoa! Turn This Horse Around

Whoa, turn that horse around. You are a spirit. You posses a soul, which is your mind, will and emotions, and you live in a physical body. You are a three-part man. The Bible says, *And God said, Let us make man in our image, after our likeness.* [Genesis 1:26] I want you to notice that God made this statement. This is not something I made up. This is not something I dreamed or is a figment of my imagination. This is what God had to say about the matter. Now I want you to see these two things:

- *And God said, Let us make man in our image and…*
- *let us make man after our likeness.*

If you study the Hebrew language, when God said, *Let us make man in our image,* He was referring to the outward appearance of God. And when He said, *let us make man after our likeness* He was referring to the inwardness of God.

And when He said, *Let us make man in our image and likeness* we know the word "our" is plural. We have a triune Godhead: there is the Father, the Son, and the Holy Spirit. It's called the Trinity. Therefore you are a three-part man: you are a spirit; you posses a soul which is your mind, will and emotions; and you live in a physical body and you have five senses.

God continues to say, *And let them have dominion over the fish of the sea, and over the fowl of the air, and over the cattle, and over all the earth, and over every creeping thing that creepeth upon the earth.* [Genesis 1:26]

I want you to notice something here. I won't cover everything specifically, but God said, "Let the man that I make or those individuals I have made (mankind which are male and female) have dominion." The word dominion simply means to dominate over. In other words, God has given mankind the ability to dominate the fish, the sea, the fowl, the cattle, anything that's on the face of the earth today. You are supposed to be able to dominate over it. God created you to have power over all things.

As a matter of the truth, Proverbs 18:21 says, *Death and life are in the power of the tongue.* I want you to get a hold of this: Death and life are in the power of *your tongue.* Do you understand what I'm saying? You have to focus on yourself in this. Someone may claim that's being selfish. No it's not. Because when you learn how to exercise the overcoming power that God has instilled on the inside of you when God made you in His image and His likeness, and when you learn how to take authority with the power God has given you, then you will be able to exercise dominion over anything and everything according to the word of God.

He said, *Let them* (male and female) *have dominion over the fish of the sea, over the fowl of the air, over the cattle, and over all the earth.* Now get a hold of that. God gave us dominion over all the earth and everything that creeps upon the earth. God made us in His image and His likeness. So when God wanted something to be a certain way, and I know this is basic, He determined what way He wanted it to be then He simply spoke it into existence. Now remember that we are made after the image and likeness of God. God patterned mankind after Himself. How can you be in the family of God and not be in the image and likeness of God? Your children resemble you, right? They're after your image and likeness. They have a few features of their own but they're basically after your image and your likeness. And we, male and female, are in the image and likeness of God Himself.

Study the scripture account of creation. When God wanted something accomplished He looked out and there was gross darkness over the face of the earth. Gross darkness. Now what did God do? If you ever want to pattern yourself after anyone, you don't have to pattern yourself after a certain kind of author, a certain kind of book, unless it's the word of God. You don't have to pattern yourself after anyone else if you'll just pattern yourself after God Himself.

> *God never spoke of the darkness. He only spoke of how He desired it to be.*

Then you will see how to operate and live in victory. We all know that in John 3:16 says that we shall not perish, and part of the meaning of the word perish means "not to lose." So it's very biblical to teach that God does not want us to lose, but wants us to win every time. To win means we have fully accomplished. If we fully accomplish then we will reach our destination or our goal or our dream in life.

When God looked out and saw gross darkness, He never spoke of the darkness. Get a hold of this. If you ever get a hold of anything in your life get a hold of this. God never spoke of the darkness. He only spoke of how He desired for it to be. In other words, He never spoke of the problem. If you pattern yourself after God, you're likely to have the God kind of success. God never spoke of what He did *not* want it to be. He only spoke of how He desired for it to be, how He wanted it to be, and therefore He said, "Light be." That's what it says in the Hebrew. It doesn't say, *Let there be light*, which is fine if you interpret it that way, but He simply said, "Light be."

You know something else I've noticed about God? He's not a man of many words. Even though He'll tell you a lot. We can take one verse out of the Bible and preach on it for a month, and yet Jesus only said maybe thirty words in that verse. Even Jesus with all the teaching He did, He was a man of few words. He got directly to the point.

So God said, "Light be." Why did He say, "Light be" when it was darkness? Because He wanted the light to appear or be here on earth. So understand that God spoke like He wanted it to be, and not the way it was, and since we were made in the image and likeness of God, so should we.

We can see this with Abraham. God taught Abraham how to do the same thing, and Abraham was able to receive and manifest the promise of God in his life. The promise of God to be the father of many nations (Genesis 12) was always available to Abraham. However, for twenty-four years his name continued to be Abram, even though the promise was available to him. And even though this promise was available to him, Abram did not understand how to develop or manifest the promise of God until God taught him how by changing his name from Abram to Abraham (Genesis 17) and by getting him to call things that were not as though they were (Romans 4:17).

You have to speak what you want it to be according to the word of God, according to the instructions of God, and according to God Himself. Now we couldn't have a better example than God Himself. I want you to keep this in mind as we're talking about getting rid of excess weight off of our bodies. We use the same principles that God taught Abraham.

You want to get rid of the excess weight off of our body and I'm showing you how to accomplish it. First, you have to learn to speak properly. You can't learn how to eat properly unless you first learn how to speak properly. You may learn how to eat properly and get rid of some weight, but you will never fully accomplish the goal without being tormented over it every day.

Do you realize that food torments people—that wrong eating torments people? I'm talking about torment. I know how it is to live in torment over food. I used to be tormented over it. When you're over 100 pounds overweight you know that something has been bugging you. That doesn't mean that I wasn't as good a person as I am now. That didn't mean that I was any less of a person than I am now. That doesn't even mean that I didn't love God as much as I do now. I just found out the secret of how to walk in victory and how to get rid of the excess weight. I didn't say *lose* it. I said to *get rid of* the excess weight and keep it off and live in victory. You do it by the words of your mouth.

The words of your mouth change the way you think. As I showed you in a previous chapter, I can take a person who doesn't want to get rid of excess weight off their body and cause them to move to the arena of "I want to" simply by the words of their mouth. You say, "You can't do that just by speaking words out of your mouth." Yes, you can do it. You can't tell me that you can't do it; I've already proven that you can.

You say, "But you had to quit eating certain things to get rid of over 100 pounds." That's exactly correct, but the way I quit eating certain foods, and the way I came to the place where I don't even desire certain foods anymore, not being a temptation anymore for me to eat the wrong foods, was through changing the way I think through my words. Changing the way you think will change your desires. You get rid of your old desires and give yourself new desires to eat what's proper and healthy for you. The new desire will cast away the old desire that wasn't good for you, and the new desire will occupy space in your mind, will, and emotions.

No two substances can occupy the same place at the same time, whether it's spiritual or physical. That's an absolute truth—a law God created. No two angels can stand in the exact same spot at the same time. I saw into the spirit world and I know it to be the truth. I've seen many angels before. You may see many in a small area, but you'll not see

Praise and encouragement will drive out discouragement.

two of them in the same place at the same time, because no two substances can occupy the same place at the same time. It is impossible.

If you have a stronghold or wrong desire in your life, and you bring in a new healthier desire and that desire is more powerful than the wrong desire, it will automatically make the wrong desire leave. It will be automatic. You don't have to make it leave; just bring the right desire on the scene and the right desire will totally replace the wrong desire because no two substances can occupy the same place at the same time. It operates the same way in the mental realm as it does in the physical.

For example, you can't think of two things at the same time, not identically at the same time. You can't do it. I will show you. Start counting to ten out loud. What's your name? You can't tell me your name and continue to count to ten. You can't do that. Your name is not "6" I don't think. Do you understand what I'm saying? You can prove it to yourself. You go look in the mirror and try to think of two things at the same time. You can think of one thing and jump over to the other, and jump back and forth, but you cannot think of two things at the same time.

I'm going to tell you something else. I'm going to get personal with you. You cannot give praise and encouragement to yourself and experience discouragement at the same time. Praise and encouragement will drive out discouragement. The only reason people don't achieve a new way of eating and getting rid of the excess weight is because of discouragement—you get talked into quitting. You have great power on the inside of you and you cannot be defeated in any area of life unless you quit.

Say, "Whoa" to the Horse

I want you to see what I'm talking about concerning your words. The title of this chapter is "Turn this Horse Around." If you were riding a horse, and you wanted to turn the horse around you'd have to get him to whoa to stop first wouldn't you? Unless you get him to make a big circle, you would have to make him stop before he could go in the opposite direction. And the word of God tells us here that you control a horse by controlling his head, by controlling his mouth with a bit and reins for direction. You have to have reins for direction. Let's look at James 3:1-5:

My brethren, be not many masters, knowing that we shall receive the greater condemnation. For in many things we offend all. If any man offend not in word, the same is a perfect man, and able also to bridle the whole body. Behold, we put bits in the horses' mouths, that they may obey us; and we turn about their whole body. Behold also the ships, which though they be so great, and are driven of fierce winds, yet are they turned about with a very small helm, whithersoever the governor listeth. Even so the tongue is a little member, and boasteth great things. Behold, how great a matter a little fire kindleth!

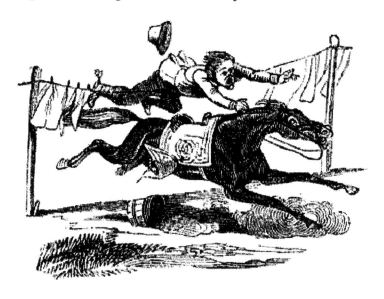

Verse 2, is what I want to show you. It says, *For in many things we offend all. If any man offend not in word, the same is a perfect*

man, and able also to bridle the whole body. That statement cannot be any more plain. It's not my interpretation, and I don't need a scholar to figure it out for me. I looked it up in the Greek and it says the same thing, but I don't need someone else's interpretation

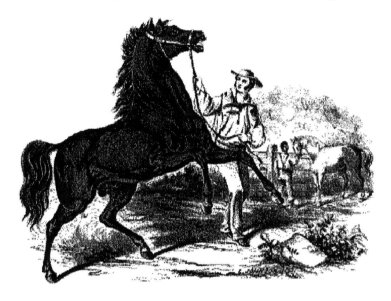

to help you out. It says that *If any man offend not in word, the same is a perfect man.*

I would say if perfect means anything close to what you think it means, it would have to be good, wouldn't it? *The same is a perfect man.* Saying he is perfect means that man is complete, or that man or woman accomplishes what the word means. The Bible goes on to say, *And they are able also to bridle the whole body.* A perfect man who does not offend in word is able to bridle or control, or lead his whole body in the direction he wants.

Because this is true, then a perfect man who controls the words of his mouth can also control his whole body and get rid of all the excess weight that's on it. This passage is talking about the words of your mouth. If you look up the word "mouth" it means "gash in the face, opening in the earth, or front edge as of a weapon."

Your mouth is a weapon. Now you can take a weapon and you can use it on your behalf. For example, if you were hungry you

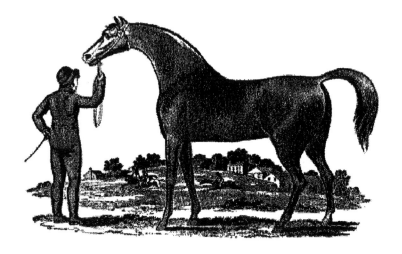

could take a weapon and go out and kill a deer and you'd have food to eat and be nourished. Or you could also take a weapon and use it against yourself. A weapon's benefit will be according to how you use it and if you use the weapon your mouth properly it will always be for you and not against you. If you use your mouth properly you will stop discouragement, which is one of the main reasons that people to fail to reach their final destination of getting rid of excess weight. The word of God says that if you can control your mouth, you are able to bridle your whole body.

Verse 3 begins, *Behold*, which means to look or to look intensely. The Lord is telling you how to control your whole body, using the way we control a horse as an example. *Behold we put bits in the horses' mouths.* Why do you put a bit in a horse's mouth? It's used to control that horse. We have learned that we can control the horse by its head, and its head with a bridle and a bit. We then use reins that are attached to each side of the bit to guide the horse where we want it to go. Reins function as a governor or driver, and since you are the governor of your body, it will go where you tell it to go. If you tell your body what and how to eat, over a period of time your body will get in tune with your mouth, your mind, and your thinking.

At the beginning of this book, we talked about the meaning of the word "diet." One of *Webster's Dictionary's* definitions of diet is "what you regularly read and think about daily." That's not the complete definition, but only a part of it. What you read, talk, think about will dictate what you

> *If you tell your body what and how to eat, over a period of time your body will get in tune with your mouth...*

eat. Not only will it dictate what you eat it, will also dictate what you desire to eat.

I'm totally convinced you will not quit eating chocolate cake for very long if you continue to tell yourself how much you like it while trying to deprive yourself of it. That's the reason that most alcoholics and food addicts do not get free. I was addicted to sweets and ate up to seven sweets and six sodas per day. I was never free until I knew the truths I'm sharing with you in this book. I went for periods of time—two or three weeks—without eating sweets, but I would always return to eating them.

I haven't eaten any sweets in years. I don't want them. I don't desire them. You may ask, "What about Thanksgiving and Christmas?" No big deal, what do Thanksgiving and Christmas have to do with eating sweets? I love Thanksgiving and Christmas. They are great holidays, but I still don't eat sweets.

Some of you may say, "Well I don't want to be where I don't eat sweets at all." That's good for someone who's not an addict. But if you were an addict like I was, you would know how strongly I was controlled and tormented by the addiction. For example, if you knew an alcoholic who was hooked on beer and you got him to where he didn't drink any beer for a period of time, you wouldn't pat him on the back and say, "Okay, go get a six-pack of beer now, you've done well." Nobody in the world would do that.

You have to be watchful in every diet plan you start. Most of them want you to *lose* the weight, but they also want you to *find* it again so you'll have to come back to them so you can *lose* it again. I'm telling you the truth. That's their objective. They can't make money from you if you don't have to keep coming back. If you got free forever and taught someone else how to be free and they told someone else and so on, the companies that create diet plans would go broke. The supply would dry up according to the demand. That's a law of economics.

A diet plan <u>should not</u> tell a person to reward himself with part of his problem. That would be like rewarding the alcoholic with a drink. Not many people can control themselves enough to just eat a little bit. Most people who are excessively overweight are that way for a reason—they don't have a lot of control in that area of their life. I was the same way before I knew the truth. I didn't drink. I didn't run around with women. I didn't do many other things, but I did have a problem controlling myself when it came to eating. Do you understand what I'm saying?

Behold, we put bits in the horses' mouth that they may obey us; and we turn about their whole body. The Lord is talking about your body. The objective is not to teach you how to control a horse; the objective is to show you how to control your body. Who will your body obey when you do it right? You. According to the word of God, control of the mouth causes your body to obey and turn around. That's when we say, "Whoa, horse. Turn around." For you, it's "Whoa, turn that body around. Start going the other way. Start living in health. Start eating properly and you will get rid of that excess weight off your body."

In verse 4, the Lord uses another example to help us understand how to control our bodies: *Behold also the ships, which though they be so great, and are driven of fierce winds, yet are they turned about with a very small helm, whithersoever the governor listeth.* You know there are fierce winds that will come against you. But did you know once you know the truth concerning proper ways of eating and getting rid of excess weight off your body, you can reach a calm place where fierce winds aren't fighting against you anymore?

If you do it right and control your tongue, you'll get rid of the temptation. I know because I've done it. There are other areas in my life I have overcome and they're not any temptation to me at all. Every person reading this book can look back in their life and find areas where they have overcome a bad habit that controlled them over a period of time and now they are not tempted in that area anymore.

I used to smoke three packs of cigarettes a day, but now I'm not tempted to smoke. Why? Because I have no desire to smoke. It is not a desire in my mind, will or emotions now to smoke cigarettes. How did that happen? A new desire has arrived and it drove out the old desire; and when it's not a desire anymore you won't be tempted by it. The Bible says that temptation occurs when a man is drawn away of his own desires and enticed (James 1:14). If the desire is not present, then there is nothing of which to draw away.

There may be a rare occasion when I have a thought to smoke a cigarette, and even then it's not a temptation. I just laugh. If you can laugh at it and not even have to send it on its way, then it's not much of a temptation, is it?

So we see that you control whatever your body does, and wherever it goes. As a ship has a captain (the Bible calls him a governor) to control the boat's direction, you are the governor of your ship, which is your body. *Behold also the ships, which though they be so great, and are driven by fierce winds, yet are they turned about with a very small helm, whithersoever the governor listeth.*

Where does that ship go? Wherever the governor desires it to go. The word *listeth* means desires. The ship or your body goes wherever you desire. A governor is the one who governs or rules over a thing. You are the ruler over your own body wherever you desire for it to go, that's where it will go.

I want to go back to verse 2 of this passage: *For in many things we offend all. And if any man offend not in word, the same is a perfect man, and he is able to bridle the whole body.* I want you to see this. The phrase *offend not in word* means that we do not fail in our words or our conversation. In other words, if we do not err or sin, or if we do not come up short or stumble in our words, then we are perfect, able to control our whole body. The more perfect you become with the words of your mouth concerning eating properly and getting rid of excess weight, then you will not offend yourself in the words that come out of your mouth.

Everyone understands that words can offend your neighbor, your wife or your family, but few understand that they can also offend you. By your words you can be encouraged or by your words you can be discouraged. Your words can cause you to have power to press through and win, or your words can bring discouragement and cause your to quit and come up short. It's the simple words of your mouth. You can take the words of your mouth, and they will become the meditations of your heart, mind, will and emotions. After you say it enough, you will begin to meditate on it, and you can move from "I don't want to" to "I want to" to "I can" to "I will" to "I am."

The words of your mouth will bring you into a perfect or complete person, and it will cause you to lack absolutely nothing.

When you move into the arena of "I am" you have now created a deep desire in your heart and you cannot be turned away. Remember that you are created in the image and likeness of God.

If you *offend not in word*, it means you will not strive against yourself. You will not strike out at yourself. You will not break the spiritual laws that cause you to win and overcome. You will not err.

You will not create resentment in yourself. You will not be angry with yourself. You will not offend yourself. You will not hurt your feelings. And if you don't hurt your own feelings then your feelings will now line up with the words of your mouth and will cause you to win and get rid of the excess weight.

This also means that you will not insult yourself. Many times a person insults themselves with their own words. You look in the mirror and call yourself fat and ugly. You should look in the mirror and tell yourself that you are the right size and you eat the proper foods to get rid of the excess weight.

According to the word of God, you body will begin to line up with the words of your mouth. Will this happen in a day or two? Not likely. But let me ask you a question: Is it worth three months of your life– ninety days of your life—for you to know that you're going to get on the road to victory and not lose? Certainly it is.

Most people jump into a diet plan out of a fleshly desire instead of preparing themselves before they ever start the diet. If you prepare yourself first with the words of your mouth and the meditations of your heart and your thinking, then you will achieve and win. The results will be that all the excess weight would just automatically come off of your body, because if you eat right, it will come off. You don't have to make it.

Now I say this not to offend anyone, but you don't need a pill to accomplish your goal of weight loss. If you use a pill to help, that's your business. I'm not trying to discourage you from taking a pill. I'm just telling you that the Bible doesn't say to use the words of your mouth and a pill. You don't have to use a powder. Some of these solutions may be good for you. I'm not a doctor. I'm just a man who knows the truth and has been set free and have lost over 100 pounds to prove it.

You do not have to have an operation to get rid of the excess weight off your body. If you do, that's your business. You don't even have to exercise. You should exercise; it's good for you to exercise, but you don't have to exercise to get rid of excess weight off your body. I got rid of 110 pounds and did absolutely no more exercise than I did before. Exercise is good for you, but God's word doesn't tell you to change the words of your mouth and exercise. You don't have to take a pill; you don't have to mix a powder; you don't have to have an operation; you don't have to exercise; and you don't need a gimmick. You just need to change the words of your mouth, the thoughts of your mind and the meditations of your heart to line up with the final destination and the word of God. God Himself says that with your words you will turn your whole body around and the excess weight will just come off.

The Bible says that when you do not offend yourself with your words, it begins to affect your taste and your senses. Your words cause you not to transgress or violate; they cause you to not have displeasure and resentment by wounding your feelings. That's what this passage is teaching. Regardless of whether your words are intentional or unintentional, wrong words will wound your feelings. They will breach or stop your prosperity or your achievement of your goal. If you speak the right words, you will not trip, you will not fail, you will not offend and you will not stumble.

The Bible says that you will be perfect. Perfection means completeness. You will be complete in getting rid of the excess weight off your body. When you become complete mentally, then your mind is not tormenting you or giving you a problem about it. Wrong foods will not be a problem for you anymore. Being perfect means you've come to full perfect character. The words of your mouth will bring you into a perfect or complete person, and it will cause you to lack absolutely nothing. It will cause you to be fully supplied.

And then the Lord says that you will be able to bridle the whole body. You have the power, and you have the capability; it is possible, and you now have the strength. You're going to bridle your whole body. You will harness your body for the purpose of guiding it in the proper direction. "Whoa, turn that horse around."

For a horse, a bit controls or restrains the body. So like a bit to the horse, the words of your mouth control or restrain your whole body. They control your destination and purpose. When you speak them properly, your words will apply pressure so that the wrong thing will automatically leave your life.

In closing this chapter, I want you to see this: I told you before that the word "mouth" is the front edge as of a weapon. Let's use that weapon against our problem and not against ourselves. Let's use that weapon against wrong food choices instead of using it the wrong way and telling ourselves that we like things that are not good for us. You might say, "Well I do like things that are not good for me."

Of course you do. That's the reason you need to change. There was darkness here and God said, "Light be." He called it the way He wanted it to be. God spoke to it the way it's supposed to be. Your mouth is the front edge of a weapon to use for your benefit and not against yourself. And once you begin speaking the right words, God's word says that your whole body will obey you. When you use the words of your mouth properly your whole body will carry out the instructions you give it.

This truth is right here in black and white. Go to the Word of God and see for yourself. Your whole body will automatically carry out the instructions you give it. You'll guide your body the right way; you'll cause it to submit; you'll bring it under control, and you will definitely turn it around. It will obey you. You will convince your body to be obedient to you. Your body will agree and give evidence of the words of your mouth. You'll begin to rely on what's true inside you, which means that your mind, will and emotions will line up with the words of your mouth.

Create a New Image

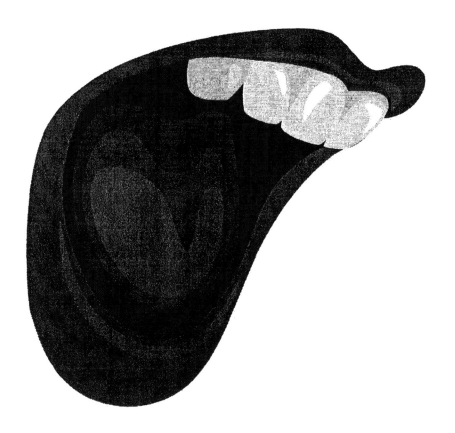

chapter
7
Create a New Image

I want to talk to you about creating a new image of yourself. The word of God says that you have the power to create. You will serve or obey the images that are in the realm of your mind, will, and emotions every day of your life. That's how you live your life on a daily basis because you see yourself in certain ways. I'm not talking about the natural image you see in the mirror, but you have certain images of yourself and that's what you follow on a daily basis. That is absolutely true.

In this chapter, I will show you how to tear down and totally destroy wrong images of yourself. I mean totally disintegrate them, and bring them to nothing. In other words, you won't just bring them down a little bit like cutting the grass and then having to cut it again a week later. What I'm talking about doing is actually uprooting a stronghold that's in your life—the stronghold of eating wrong foods. You will actually take that stronghold by the roots and tear it out.

I want you to know that you cannot accomplish spiritual things by operating in the flesh, or by warring in the flesh. The word of God says, *For though we walk in the flesh, we do not war after the flesh: (For the weapons of our warfare are not carnal, but mighty through God to the pulling down of strong holds;) Casting down imaginations, and every high thing that exalteth itself against the knowledge of God, and bringing into captivity every thought to the obedience of Christ.* [2 Corinthians 10:3-5]

Because the correct image of yourself is spiritual, you cannot create a new image on the inside of you by doing it out of the flesh. You have to move into the spiritual realm to be able to accomplish it. It is accomplished by the words of your mouth and by the thoughts and the meditations of your heart. You accomplish this by building new images.

Let us remember that no two substances can occupy the same place at the same time. Do not be deceived – everyone has an image of himself that was developed from his imagination. God created you with an imagination and the ability to form images. Having an imagination is not a bad thing. God created you that way. The images you create in that realm can be either good or bad.

With those thoughts in mind, please understand you cannot tear down the stronghold of false or negative images in your imagination by the flesh. You cannot do it. People try and do it all the time. I said this in a previous chapter where people always want to start on a diet from the "want to" realm, just because they say, "I want to." "I want to" is a good starting place but that is not a finishing place, and you cannot reach your goal by staying in the "want to" realm, because the "want to" realm is the fleshly realm.

How many things do you have in your life right now that you would like to get rid of or lay down? In this book, we're talking about wrong eating habits, but you can utilize these principles with anything in life. How many wrong eating habits do you have that are not good for you? All of them have been created in you through your imagination and this is the image you have of yourself, which is the

You cannot pull down a stronghold in your life by agreeing with it.

reason you haven't been able to lay it down or get rid of it permanently. The word permanently means forever—to never return again. If it's permanent, it's not for a day or two or a week or a month or even just for a year. If it's permanent, it's forever.

104

I'm talking about getting rid of things forever, casting them out of you life, and tearing down these false images that have been created on the inside of you. You created these images. Maybe you had help from other people, but you created them by the words of your mouth and by the meditations of your mind or your heart. You cannot get rid of them through the flesh. You must get rid of them through the spirit and the words of your mouth. Your words are spiritual and they are so powerful that they carry life or they carry death. The miracle working power that lies on the inside of you comes out of your mouth and your heart.

So then, the Bible says that we cannot accomplish this by warring after the flesh. It says that *the weapons of our warfare are not carnal* (not of the flesh) *but mighty through God to the pulling down of strong holds.* You have to learn how to pull down that stronghold. The word stronghold is interpreted as imagination or image. Therefore, you must learn how to pull down these strongholds, not from the natural or flesh realm but from the spiritual realm.

You pull down strongholds <u>not</u> by agreeing with them but by disagreeing with them. You cannot pull down a stronghold in your life by agreeing with it. A person who agrees they have no self-control will always submit to this statement because it is an image they have of themselves. A person who agrees he has no self-control, but yet tries to control himself has defeated himself before the battle begins. He may resist for a time, but at the end, he will always revert back to the image he has for himself. You may have a stronghold of thinking you're not good enough. Many people have strongholds like that. Did you know that having a negative image causes people to eat wrong foods? People who have a negative image of themselves often believe they cannot change as well. As long as you think you can't change then you won't. You must convince yourself that you can change; and not only that you *can* change, but you *will* change.

So we have to pull down these strongholds. When it says to

pull down strongholds it means to cast them down and demolish them. It means to demolish those bad imaginations or images. That's all a stronghold is: a bad or negative image that has been created on the inside of you. A stronghold has a *strong hold* in your life because it has deep roots in your soul: your mind, will and emotions. It has deep roots and therefore it's always looking for a food source. The only way a stronghold gets its food source or nourishment is by getting you to agree with the negative image and speaking the same way. Every time you line your mouth up with the negative image, you are feeding the negative image and keeping it alive.

Therefore, in order to demolish or destroy the negative image of wrong food choices then you must not feed it anymore through your words. You cannot continue to say that you like certain kinds of food while at the same time, try to refrain from eating them. You must starve the stronghold, you must deteriorate it, and pull it down with the power of your words by telling yourself that you do not like those foods anymore.

This works not only in your eating lifestyle, but also with any problem, addiction, or bad habit in your life. Don't ever tell yourself how poorly you think of yourself and that you can't do any better, using the excuse that this is just the way you are. That way of thinking is an excuse from the pit of hell. Let me be honest with you. You can do better and the power to do better is right on the inside of you. All you have to do is line up your thinking and mouth with the truths I've been sharing in this book. If you think and talk the right way, not only can you do better, but you will do better.

When you pull down a stronghold, you're going to demolish, extinguish, and weaken it until it disappears. You're not going to support it anymore. Think about that. You need to tell yourself, "I will not support wrong eating habits with the words of my mouth. I will never tell myself again that I like chocolate cake." Whatever your problem may be, you must not agree and support this problem with your words.

For me, I tell myself that I hate chocolate cake, and because of this confession, I haven't desired a piece of it in two and a half years. I don't even want it anymore. I don't smoke for the same reason. I quit smoking thirty years ago and I don't want them anymore. It's not hard to resist something when you don't want it anymore. It's easy to resist eating sweets when you don't want them anymore.

I have actually changed the desires of my heart, mind, will and emotions. Now I don't even desire it. It's not a problem to stay away from something when you don't want it. Think of a food that you don't like: it is not difficult for you to refuse to eat that food. Because you don't like it, and don't want it, you're not even tempted to eat it. When you continue to tell yourself and bring yourself to the point that you don't like and don't want to eat the wrong food, then it will not be a temptation anymore.

To be strong means to be physically powerful; having great strength; not easily affected or upset. In other words, you'll be strong in these areas. You're going to cast and pull it down. If you'll study the word stronghold, it refers to a castle that has walls built around it. The words of your mouth have built walls around a false image or around a castle in your life that came out of your imagination. This is a stronghold in your soul and it can be torn down the same way it was built.

You were not born with this image in you. It had to be

> *It's not hard to resist something when you don't want it anymore.*

created in you over a period of time. Other people—your parents for example, may have helped, but you had to finish building it. I have told you this before and I'm going to tell you again: You don't believe anyone as much as you believe yourself.

A stronghold is a place having a strong defense; it's a fortified place; a place that has been made strong physically and emotionally. Walls have been built around it. A stronghold affects your views—the way you see things and it also affects your attitude. It affects everything about you.

I told you previously that no two substances could occupy the same place at the same time. Therefore, you're going to tear down negative images that you have of yourself: thinking that you cannot do any better, that you cannot achieve, that you cannot get rid of the excess weight, that you always fail when you go on a diet. Remember that you're already on a diet; everybody is on one. It may be a good healthy one, or it may be one that's not good for you. It may be one that takes off the excess weight from your body, or it may be one that puts excess weight on your body. And all you have to do is reverse it. All you have to do is change it.

The way that you tear down these false images is by doing the opposite of how you built them, which was through your words. You're going to tear them down by speaking the opposite of the image. Whatever the image tells you in your mind's eye you simply speak the opposite of it. You do as God would do and "call things that be not as though they were." Declare that you're already free, that you already have the right way of travel and then you are going to create a new image on the inside of you.

You are going to create a new image on the inside of you and this is a new image that has never existed before. And you know that it has never existed before because of your past failures. How many times have you tried new diet plans and stayed on them for a week or a month or for so long but did not accomplish your final mission? How many times? The reason you didn't accomplish and get the excess weight off your body is because you failed to create a new image to take the place of the old image.

At the same time you are creating a new image, you're also tearing down the old image. When the new image emerges, the old image has to leave and then you'll begin to follow the new image that you have created. Through the words of your mouth, you can be free of wrong eating and excess weight or you can be free of anything that would destroy your body.

I'm talking about being totally free, not barely getting by, but being completely unrestrained, and not being pressured anymore. So when you begin creating this new image, it means that you are going to cause it to grow. Every word that comes out of your mouth is a seed, and every seed brings forth a crop. Words are containers and words are full of substance. The seeds will start creating this new image that you desire to be.

Words will automatically create it because that's the way God made you and designed you after Himself. In the same way that God created the worlds with the words of His mouth, and saw that it was good, you too will see that it's good. How many of you know that good is not bad. Some young folks call bad things "good" and good things "bad" but let me tell you good is good.

If you ever do a real research on the word good, you'll find out that this word is the most accurate word you can use to describe God. When you go into the Greek and the Hebrew, you'll find out that it's not "good, better, and best" like it is in the English language. The truth is that the word "good" is the best and better. The word of God says that God is good, and you can't get any closer to God than good. Good is the ultimate.

Therefore, when you create a good (or godly) image on the inside of yourself, then you will follow that good image and it will not be hard. You must understand this! If you've ever heard anything in your life, then hear me now. It won't be hard. If you spend time creating a new image on the inside of yourself, then you will not struggle and strain trying to accomplish it like you have in the past.

What does it mean to create? It means, "to cause to grow; to cause to come into existence." By the words of your mouth, you're going to cause a new image on the inside of you to come into existence. All you have to do is open your mouth and say it. You might say, "I don't even believe it." It doesn't matter.

No person automatically begins believing this. You have to get to the point of believing it. Whether you believe it or not, after you say it for a certain length of time, you'll eventually begin to think about what you're saying and it'll catch up with you. Then, after you begin to think about, meditate, ponder and study on what you're saying, it won't be too long before you'll start believing what you say. In order for these truths to work, you must believe it. I'm not eliminating the fact that you must exercise faith in order to accomplish your goal. You must believe, and your results will be according to your faith. However, because these truths seem to be unusual to your natural mind, you have to get to the point of believing it. And this comes through words because *faith cometh by hearing, and hearing by the word of God.* [Romans 10:17] Faith comes by hearing words.

Repetition of God's word is good and will produce the results you desire. You have to hear it over and over again.

I remember when my wife was first told about Jesus, she did not believe in Him. But they kept telling her how much God loved her and kept on and on and on and on. And after she heard it so much, she finally began to believe it. No one starts off believing anything. If you believed from day one that you could overcome the problem of wrong eating and excess weight on your body, you would have already overcome it.

No one starts off at the top of the ladder as an expert. You may have a talent, but you still have to be trained. You still have to de disciplined. Do you hear what I'm saying? So when you continue to tell yourself that you like these good food choices and you do not like the wrong food choices, before long you will convince yourself.

Think about the word "convince." Did you know that "convince" is a part of the word "faith"? Faith is being able to convince. It's confidence. No one starts off with confidence, but through your words, you begin to gain confidence that you can and will and are achieving the final goal. Faith and confidence are identical. They work hand in hand. They're twins. If you have faith, then you have confidence. If you have confidence, then you have faith.

Romans 10:17 says that faith or confidence (they are interchangeable) comes by hearing the word of God over a period of time. Repetition of the word of God is good and will produce the results you desire. You have to hear it over and over again. Therefore, when you repeatedly tell yourself, you'll gain confidence and get to the point where you will create a new image. You will bring it into being, make it, and originate something that did not exist before.

You're going to bring about this new image on the inside of you. You're going to give rise to it. It will be the highlight of your life concerning food and food choices. You will cause it to be. You are inventing it. You will bring it to a new realm or a new rank in life. You will create a new image. All you have to do is to renew your mind to that image you want on the inside of you.

If this is to be a new image that never existed before, it will appear initially and develop in your imagination. It will be produced for the first time in your life. It will manifest and it will always bring forth fruit—always. You will have new understanding of the problem that you used to have. You'll begin to see why you had that problem of wrong eating for all of those years. You don't have to worry about getting rid of excess weight off your body; all you have to do is make smarter food choices and excess weight will leave. You won't have to be concerned about excess weight, it will just leave your body. Excess weight never belonged to you to start with. It was not part of you.

Did you know that bad habits and wrong things in your life

are really not part of you? They are things that have been added to you. You weren't conceived having a nicotine habit. You weren't conceived with a drug or alcohol habit. Think about it. It had to be added to you either by your mother in the womb (in the case of babies being born with drug addictions) or through your personal choices. You had to develop it. You had to get an image of yourself that way. The reason people don't lay down things that they ought to lay down and walk away from is because they have an image of it inside them—they can't see themselves without it.

At first this will be strange to you. Have you ever met a new person? At first they seemed a little strange because you weren't used to being around them. But the more you hung around them, the more acquainted and comfortable you become. It's just like going to a new church. It might be a little strange to you at first, but the more you go, the more you become acquainted with it. You can't tell in one or two visits. You've got to hang around a while.

It's the same way with creating a new image on the inside of you concerning right food habits and right food choices. Once you get acquainted with these truths, the more you can befriend them and understand them. At first it will seem strange—like it's not real. It'll seem uncomfortable—like it's not really true—but I guarantee you by a promise from God Himself that if you will continue to say it, then sooner or later you will befriend this new image, and become associated with it, and it will actually become a part of you. You're making another start of getting rid of excess weight off your body, but this time you're doing it the right way. You're doing it with quality and with vigor and most importantly, you're doing it God's way.

I want to talk to you about the image—about creating the new one and destroying the old one. What is an image? An image is a visual impression of something that is produced from a mental picture. That's exactly what it is. I'll repeat that: an image is a visual impression of something that is produced from a mental picture. Think about a painter. The artist has an image in their mind what he or she wants to portray on the canvas. Therefore, every painting is an image of what was conceived first in the artist's mind. It is a conception; it is an idea. An image is an impression. Isn't that amazing?

You're building fresh concepts on the inside of you. Let me tell you what a concept is. A concept is an idea or a thought, an abstract motion. Some concepts are not easy to understand in the beginning, but through repetition, they become a way of life. The concept becomes reality. It takes away the old and builds the new. It's like conceiving an embryo or a fetus that is actually born on the inside of you.

The word of God says that a man's belly or a man's womb (his spiritual reproductive place) shall be satisfied with the fruit of his mouth. And then it goes on to say that death and life are in the power of the tongue (Proverbs 18:20-21). You've experienced death, not by falling over dead, but you destroyed yourself by having excess weight on your body by making wrong food choices. You can also experience life through your words.

Death and life are in the power of the tongue, the *dunamis*, miracle-working power of the tongue. This is not easy to understand at first, but once you continue, it becomes a way of life. That which is conceived, like an embryo, is the beginning of a process or change of events. Words, thoughts and ideas formulate the image. It is an expressed plan in a systematic way with the (dunamis) miracle-working power of God by the words of your mouth.

An image is a visual impression of something that is produced from a mental picture.

You will form this new image in your mind and develop it. You formulate building this new image on the inside of you. It is a mental impression, an original design. You have to start seeing yourself as an overcomer, a victor, as getting rid of bad eating habits and excess weight off your body that does not belong to you. The image you form is one where you see yourself eating proper foods, and this is accomplished by telling yourself how much you like these proper foods. Even if you don't feel like it, tell yourself anyway, and it will cause you to get rid of the excess weight from your body.

Like the bit and bridle to a horse's body, your words control and dictate your body. The old wrong habits no longer control and dictate you. You have now built a new image, a new image on the inside of you that you're following. The old image is cast out, torn down; it is brought to nothing and it doesn't dictate your life anymore. Your life is now dictated by the new image you have built on the inside of you. Start seeing yourself as an overcomer, a victor.

You control your body and your soul: your mind, will, and emotions. Your body and soul were given to you by God to be a servant, to serve you and it will serve good or bad. All the soul knows how to do is to serve. Like a computer, all it knows how to do is to operate according to its programming. Your soul only knows how to serve and it will serve good or bad according to what's programmed in it.

Remember the passage from James that says that you are the governor. You are the captain of your mind, will and emotions and body, and you steer them with your words. They are now obeying and listening to you. New programming is taking place, developing a new image on the inside of you and all rebellion is gone.

Creating a new image is not accomplished in the flesh. You a have to pull down those strongholds and build new images with your words, which is a more powerful weapon. Your words and meditations will uproot deeply rooted images that were created in the imagination. Tell yourself day and night and you will begin to believe and you will create the new image on the inside and you will follow that new image.

Don't ever think you have to remain in the old pattern of life, because you don't. You can be transformed by the renewing and reprogramming of your mind. Through these truths, you can bring completeness to yourself. That's the way you do it. The word of God says that when you renew your mind, you will prove and give visible evidence that it works every time.

And be not conformed to this world; but be ye transformed by the renewing of your mind, that ye may prove what is that good, and acceptable, and perfect will of God. [Romans 12:2]

Please contact us for additional help and materials regarding *Fat Free Forever.*

Pastor/Evangelist Bobby Ray teaches many other subjects and has numerous materials available for help and guidance.

To book Bobby Ray for speaking engagements and other events please call 704.922.9701.

We are here to serve you so you can move forward in life in a positive light. We welcome your inquiries!

Bobby Ray Ministries
P.O. Box 1092
Dallas, NC 28034
704.922.9701 or 704.629.0394
brminalive@aol.com
www.bobbyray.org